Mediterranean Diet Meal Prep 2020

Practical Guide With over 40 recipes, 4 Weekly Meals, 10 Tips For Your Success, To Lose Weight In Healthy Way Saving Time and Money.

Elisa Rossi

© Copyright 2020 - All rights reserved.

The content contained within this book may not be reproduced, duplicated or transmitted without direct written permission from the author or the publisher.

Under no circumstances will any blame or legal responsibility be held against the publisher, or author, for any damages, reparation, or monetary loss due to the information contained within this book, either directly or indirectly.

Legal Notice:

This book is copyright protected. It is only for personal use. You cannot amend, distribute, sell, use, quote or paraphrase any part, or the content within this book, without the consent of the author or publisher.

Disclaimer Notice:

Please note the information contained within this document is for educational and entertainment purposes only. All effort has been executed to present accurate, up to date, reliable, complete information. No warranties of any kind are declared or implied. Readers acknowledge that the author is not engaged in the rendering of legal, financial, medical or professional advice. The content within this book has been derived from various sources. Please consult a licensed professional before attempting any techniques outlined in this book.

By reading this document, the reader agrees that under no circumstances is the author responsible for any losses, direct or indirect, that are incurred as a result of the use of the information contained within this document, including, but not limited to, errors, omissions, or inaccuracies.

Thanks for choosing this book, make sure to leave a short review on Amazon if you enjoy it. I'd really love to hear your thoughts.

Summary

Introduction 9

Chapter 1: Understanding the Mediterranean Diet 12

    Health Benefits 13

    Disadvantages of the Mediterranean Diet 16

Chapter 2: Eating the Mediterranean Way 20

    Mediterranean Food Pyramid 21

    Food Lists 25

    Cleaning out Your Cupboards 29

Chapter 3: Your Meal Planning Guide 32

    Getting Started on Your Meal Plan 33

    From Meal Planning to Meal Prepping 36

    Organizing Your Meal Plan 37

    Sticking to Your Budget 40

Chapter 4: Your Grocery Shopping Guide 43

    Before You Go Shopping 43

    Tips to Give You the Best Shopping Experience 44

    Creating Your Grocery List 46

Chapter 5: Week One Meal Plan 50

    Monday 51

    Tuesday 51

    Wednesday 52

    Thursday 53

    Friday 53

    Saturday 54

Sunday 55

Chapter 6: Week Two Meal Plan 57

Monday 57

Tuesday 57

Wednesday 58

Thursday 58

Friday 59

Saturday 59

Sunday 60

Chapter 7: Week Three Meal Plan 62

Monday 62

Tuesday 62

Wednesday 63

Thursday 63

Friday 64

Saturday 64

Sunday 65

Chapter 8: Week Four Meal Plan 67

Monday 67

Tuesday 67

Wednesday 68

Thursday 68

Friday 69

Saturday 69

Sunday 70

Chapter 9: Mediterranean Recipes 73

Breakfast 73
- Greek Quinoa Breakfast Bowl.. 73
- Bulgur Fruit Breakfast Bowl 74
- Coconut and Banana Mix 75
- Honey Nut Granola 77
- Cheese and Cauliflower Frittata With Peppers............ 78
- Omelet With Cheese and Broccoli........................... 80
- Almond Pancakes 81
- Pear and Mango Smoothie 83
- Egg-Artichoke Breakfast Casserole 84
- Breakfast Burrito Mediterranean Style 86
- Ham and Egg Muffins 87
- Thick Pomegranate Cherry Smoothie 88

Lunch 89
- Delicious Broccoli Tortellini Salad........................... 89
- Grilled Lemon Fish 91
- Chicken Drummies With Peach Glaze 92
- Mediterranean Potato Salad 94
- Bean Lettuce Wraps 95
- Tuna Bowl With Kale 97
- Italian Tuna Sandwiches 98
- Flatbread With Roasted Vegetables 99
- Steamed Mussels Topped With Wine Sauce............. 101
- Carrot Soup With Parmesan Croutons 103

Dinner 105
- Spinach and Beans Mediterranean Style Salad......... 105

Lasagna 106

Salmon Skillet Dinner 109

Barley and Mushroom Soup 110

Seafood Paella 112

Italian Baked Beans 114

Chickpeas and Brussel Sprouts Salad 115

Vegetarian Lasagna Roll-Ups 116

Mediterranean Pizza 118

Garlic and Cajun Shrimp Bowl With Noodles 120

Grilled Calamari With Berries 121

Dessert 122

Chocolate Fruit Kebabs 122

A Lemony Treat 124

Cherry Brownies With Walnuts 126

Stuffed Figs 127

Melon With Ginger 128

Chia Pudding With Strawberries 129

Peaches With Blue Cheese Cream 130

Mediterranean Blackberry Ice Cream 131

Almond Shortbread Cookies 133

Fruit Dip 134

Snacks 135

Baked Apples Mediterranean Style 135

Fig-Pecan Energy Bites 136

Frozen Blueberry Yogurt 137

Strawberry Popsicle 138

Chunky Monkey Trail Mix 139

Chapter 10: Ten Tips for Success **142**

Tip 1: Be Proud of Yourself Everyday 142

Tip 2: Focus on Controlling Your Portions.................. 143

Tip 3: Make Time in Your Schedule to Focus on Your Meal Plan 144

Tip 4: Write Down Your Ideas................................. 145

Tip 5: Always Keep Staple Foods in Your Kitchen........ 146

Tip 6: Take Time to Eat.. 146

Tip 7: You Don't Need to Prepare Every Meal............. 147

Tip 8: Let Your Food Cool Down All the Way Before Freezing 148

Tip 9: Don't Skip Breakfast 148

Tip 10: Forgive Yourself 148

Conclusion **151**

Introduction

You hear about a new diet every year—sometimes more than once a year. It seems that wherever you look, you're reading about the newest and best diet around. You've thought about incorporating a diet into your life, but you're not sure which one. You want a diet where you can continue to eat some of your favorite foods, but also one that will give your taste buds a new and exciting flavor.

The origins of the Mediterranean diet are hard to find because they go back to the Middle Ages. Some people believe the diet goes back to the days of the Ancient Romans, where they would eat bread, oils, and drink wine with their meals. They also ate very little red meat, focusing more on seafood and plant-based foods. Romans ate in gluttony and didn't focus on how much food they put into their bodies. They didn't know about counting calories, fats, proteins, or any other nutrients. They ate throughout the day, sometimes meals would last a couple of hours, especially during celebrations. Needless to say, the way people follow the diet today is a bit different.

Unlike the ancient Romans, people pay attention to how much food they eat in a day. For instance, they will count their calories, protein, and fat intake. They will also limit the amount of poultry and red meat they eat. The Romans did not limit their red meats, they simply did not eat it much. The biggest difference today is that people follow a food pyramid, which tells them how much food they can have throughout the day. For example, they will eat fruits, vegetables, whole grains, herbs, or oils in every meal while eating poultry, cheese, and eggs sparingly throughout the week.

The biggest problem people have with the Mediterranean diet is that they start the diet without fully understanding the basic information, what foods to eat daily, what foods to eat sparingly, and how to develop and follow a meal plan. Without looking at ways to ensure success, failure is a bigger probability. This is the main reason I created this book. Not only do I want to give you all the basic information and make sure you understand how to eat the Mediterranean way, but I want to help you set up a meal plan. I want to walk with you through the process of starting this diet, so you are set up for success.

The first couple of chapters will focus on the basics of the Mediterranean diet. You will learn the foundation and a bit of history along with why scientists believe the diet is successful. The Mediterranean food pyramid is described along with the benefits and disadvantages that you will face. You will get a clear idea of what foods you can eat and which foods you should eat sparingly or avoid. Don't worry about how you will clean out your cupboards when it comes to starting the diet because this is discussed as well.

The middle of the book focuses on meal planning and how you will start this process. You might wonder how you'll fix healthy meals when you live such a busy life, but one fun fact about the Mediterranean diet is the meals are easy to plan and prepare, giving you an easier evening during the stressful workweeks. You will receive all the information you need to start your meal plan, such as what to include, how to stay within your budget, and how to stay organized.

I will also guide you through your first shopping experience.

Chapters 5 through 8 focus on a meal plan for your first four weeks. Throughout these chapters, you will receive a full meal plan from breakfast through dinner. The plan includes drinks to have with your meals and snack ideas for the day. A fun bonus in these few chapters is recipes. Some of the meals are easily created, such as mixing Greek yogurt with your favorite fruit for breakfast, but some meals might be newer to you or you may not be sure how to make it the Mediterranean way so I included the recipe at the end of the day.

Don't think that you'll only find recipes throughout your weekly meal plans. You will get over 40 recipes in chapter 9 that will help you stay within your budget and follow the diet.

Finally, you'll receive 10 tips for success from people who understand the Mediterranean diet and how to eat in this fashion. By following these tips, you will have no trouble staying on the right path. Of course, these tips will not take away any cravings or struggles that you'll face, especially during your first few weeks, but they will help give you the support you need.

Chapter 1: Understanding the Mediterranean Diet

The Mediterranean diet is a bit different than other types of diets. In fact, some people do not consider it a diet at all, they treat it as a new way of life or a different eating pattern. While there are some foods that you should avoid, it is not a huge list. This diet will not make you stop eating some of your favorite foods. It will not tell you to go on a juice cleanse for a few days or start by fasting so your body can start to lose weight faster. This diet is all about learning what foods are the best for you to eat. In other words, the Mediterranean diet is about eating healthy. But this is only part of what it's about. The other part is that you add a different flavor to your foods because you'll use cooking methods and focus on foods that are connected to the Mediterranean.

The basis of the diet comes from the area along the Mediterranean Sea, which is connected to the Atlantic Ocean. It's surrounded by countries like Spain, Italy, Croatia, France, Greece, Turkey, Egypt, Israel, and many other civilizations along the Mediterranean basin. The reason doctors and dieticians started to note the Mediterranean diet is because people who live along the sea live longer than Americans. Furthermore, they do not suffer from cardiovascular diseases, cancers, and other health problems as often. This is not to say that people along the sea don't get diseases. However, their statistics are much lower than American statistics and many researchers believe this is because of the food they eat.

Health Benefits

The Mediterranean diet has many health benefits, which is one of the main reasons it's become so popular. Several years ago, two professors from the Harvard School of Public Health, Dimitrios Trichopoulos who is the Vincent L. Gregory Professor of Cancer Prevention and Walter Willett, the chair for the Department of Nutrition and Fredrick John Stare Professor of Epidemiology and Nutrition, studied the Mediterranean diet and proved that not only is it a diet that provides a lot of health benefits, but it's the best diet for people to follow. According to the professors, to get the best health benefits, you need to follow all of the diet's guidelines and parts. As Professor Willett told the *Los Angeles Times* in an article, "No one part is most important. They're all important. It's the combination of all the parts that matters" ("Nutrition news: Widely studied Mediterranean diet linked to good health", n.d.).

Do you feel that your eyes are getting worse? This is a common problem that happens when people age, but many people start to lose their eyesight at a young age. While this is easily fixed through prescription glasses or contacts, this diet can help improve your eyesight. It might not bring you to a point of never needing a prescription for your sight again, but it will help you prevent macular degeneration. This disease is very common among people who are over the age of 54 and destroys your retina, which helps you see clearly. The better vision comes because of all the vegetables and fish you eat. Remember when your mother or grandmother used to tell you that carrots help you see—

she was right! Omega-3 fatty acids help reduce the risk of macular degeneration.

The enjoyment of eating foods that are natural instead of processed ones is another health benefit. Not only will you feel better overall, but you'll feel the satisfaction of taking good care of your body. You will start to focus on the foods you put into your body. The healthier you feel, the more you will want to focus on eating the Mediterranean way. Plus, you don't have to give up your favorite desserts when you start the diet.

Like most diets, the Mediterranean diet helps you lose weight. The difference between this diet and many other diets is that you are more likely to keep the pounds off. Because you focus on creating a healthy meal plan, eating healthy fats over unhealthy fats, and eat foods that are rich in nutrients, you feel more energized and it is easier for you to stay active and keep those pounds off.

The number of people with cardiovascular disease in the United States is on the rise. One of the best benefits of this diet is it will reduce your risk of heart disease and stroke. In part, this is because you'll eat foods that focus on healthy "good" cholesterol, also known as High-density lipoprotein (HDL), instead of unhealthy "bad" cholesterol or low-density lipoprotein (LDL). Foods that are processed are rich in LDL, which sticks to your arteries and clogs them.

Along with lowering the risk of cardiovascular disease, the Mediterranean diet is known to reduce the risk of Parkinson's and Alzheimer's disease. Scientific studies prove that people who eat Mediterranean based foods see a

40% reduction in risk factors for Alzheimer's disease (Berti et al., 2018). This happens because the earliest stages of the disease slow down, which allows a slower progression if the disease does start. It is important to keep people on the diet if they start to show signs of Alzheimer's Disease. The reason that Parkinson's disease is reduced focuses on the oxidative stress that the diet prevents because of the amount of antioxidants you eat. Oxidative stress causes cell damage, which impacts regions of the brain that are associated with Parkinson's Disease.

Decreased risk of diabetes is another health benefit of following the diet. Because you eat more foods that help you lose weight and lower your blood sugar levels, the fatty acids help reduce risk factors associated with diabetes. In a sense, your body becomes more balanced when it comes to your blood sugar levels, insulin levels, and weight. Plus, you become more active due to your increased energy.

If you suffer from asthma, you will want to try the Mediterranean diet. Studies show that the foods you eat help asthma symptoms because of the antioxidants that your body receives (Papamichael, Katsardis & Lambert, 2018). Plus, you eat less red meat and more plant-based foods, which will naturally help your asthma symptoms.

Disadvantages of the Mediterranean Diet

Whenever you have a list of benefits, you will also find a list of disadvantages. To give you the greatest knowledge of the diet, it is important that you understand both sides.

One of the disadvantages is that some of the food can cost a bit more than what you want to spend. Fortunately, there isn't a lot of expensive Mediterranean food, but the foods that are spendy can keep you from even trying them. You will eat a lot of seafood on your diet. Because you eat it several times a week, you will want to mix it up. While recipes will help, you still do not want to stick to tuna and fish all of the time. You will start to crave other foods, such as lobster. While lobster is a great choice, it is also one of the most expensive as you will pay about $12 to $15 per pound, depending on your location.

So, what can you do if you want some lobster but need to save money? The best tip is to watch your local grocery stores for sales and stock up on the seafood that you want when it's on sale. For example, if the grocery store is offering so much off per pound, it's time for you to go grocery shopping. The trick is to make sure you can adequately store the food at home. For example, it might be hard for you to buy a couple of live lobsters and store them in your home until you are ready to make the meal.

A second disadvantage is if you struggle with a health condition, such as diabetes or heart disease, you will need extra guidance and health check-ups to make sure that you're on the right track and the diet is helping you rather than making your condition worse. While eating the Mediterranean way is known to decrease the symptoms and chances of developing diseases, this does not mean you won't have complications if you have certain diseases and start the diet. You will eat a lot of carbohydrates on this diet, which is dangerous for people with diabetes. To make sure your blood sugar does not spike because of an unbalanced number of carbohydrates, you might consult a dietitian to help you create a meal plan that is focused on balancing your carbs and sugars. Moreover, your body changes on the diet so you might find yourself becoming sick easily, struggling with insomnia, or feeling worse overall.

Many people see drinking wine on the Mediterranean diet as more of a benefit, especially after a stressful day, but for many other people, they cannot drink alcohol or do not want to. First, it is important to realize that no one who promotes the diet is forcing anyone to drink. Second, the diet is specific when it states that you should not have more than one glass of alcohol in a day. It does state that it is fine to drink a glass of wine daily, but no more than one glass. Of course, all professionals who support the diet encourage people to follow their own beliefs and guidelines when it comes to drinking alcohol. If it's best that you do not drink, then choose a glass of water, milk, or freshly squeezed juice over wine.

A final disadvantage is the same as most diets, you will find yourself craving foods that you can only have in moderation or not at all. For example, you are to limit all red meats to 0 to 1 serving every week. If you eat red meat, such as hamburgers, steak, or pork, on a regular basis then you might struggle cutting back. The challenge of fighting off the cravings might make you feel like you cannot follow the diet, which can cause you to give in to cravings or give up on the diet. In this case, the best tip to follow is to eat a little more red meat but in smaller portions. For example, have a small sausage patty in the morning on Monday and then have another small piece of red meat on Thursday. This will split up your portion for the week and help you settle any cravings.

Notes:

Chapter 2: Eating the Mediterranean Way

Dietitians and the American Heart Association state that there are three main rules to follow when you're eating the Mediterranean way. First, you'll want to eat a plentiful amount of fruits and vegetables. They are a great source of nutrients and most are low in calories and carbohydrates. Even though the Mediterranean diet does not focus on limiting carbohydrates, most people like to keep their carb and calorie intake to a minimum. For instance, they might follow a guideline that allows them to eat only 75 grams of carbohydrates in a 1,800 calorie a day diet.

Along with fruits and vegetables, you want to eat an abundance of whole grains, legumes, and beans. If you find yourself limiting carbohydrates to the point where you're following more of a low-carb diet, then you want to look at switching to a low-carb diet or increase your carb intake on the Mediterranean diet. This diet focuses more on carbs than other diets. However, carbohydrates are a part of the healthy food groups, which allows you to lose weight, feel full longer, and gain several health benefits.

Second, you need to ensure you include fish, seafood, oils, herbs, seeds, and nuts as often as possible. Some people will include poultry in this section, but you need to eat more seafood than poultry.

Third, you need to limit the amount of red meat, processed foods, sugary beverages, and sweets that you eat. While you do not need to completely avoid these foods, though some people will, you want to keep them to 0 to 2 servings a week. It is also a good idea to never eat more than one limited item in a day. For example, if you want to have a hamburger for dinner, you shouldn't have a brownie or a can of soda on the same day.

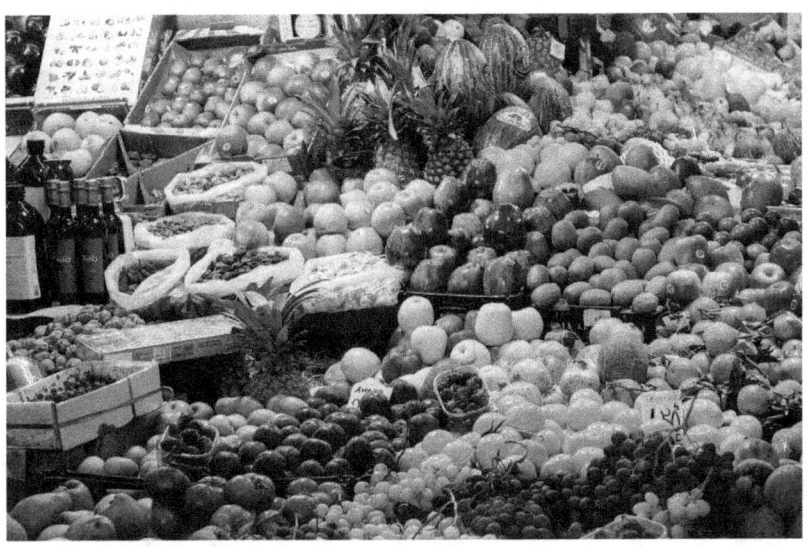

Mediterranean Food Pyramid

One of the first steps researchers took was to develop the Mediterranean Diet Pyramid, which explains what you can and cannot eat. In 1993, scientists from the European Office of the World Health Organization, Old Preservation and Exchange Trust, and the Harvard School of Public Health came together to create this pyramid to guide people interested in following the diet for health reasons ("Diet Review: Mediterranean Diet", 2018).

The most important information and foods start at the bottom of the pyramid with daily activity and spending time with family. Not only should families eat together, but they need to keep each other active, such as playing sports, riding bikes, roller skating, and walking.

Above daily activities and family time is eating enough whole-grains, beans, breads, seeds, and nuts. These are food items that you should eat every day. In fact, some people will make sure that they have food from this group with every meal. Some of the foods in this group include buckwheat, whole-grain bread, pumpkin seeds, peas, brown rice, lentils, chickpeas, barley, sesame seeds, walnuts, pasta, pine nuts, corn, almonds, cashews, macadamia nuts, hazelnuts, whole oats, and sunflower seeds. These items not only make a great snack, but they can also be incorporated into hundreds of recipes.

The next food group is fruits and vegetables. These are also considered daily foods on the diet and are eaten as snacks and meals. Some of the foods on this list include strawberries, grapes, onions, dates, peaches, carrots, figs, melons, pears, broccoli, kale, apples, tomatoes, cauliflower, Brussels sprouts, bananas, cucumbers, oranges, and spinach. Fruits and vegetables are in the same daily category, but most dietitians state you should eat more vegetables than fruits. In fact, many pyramids show that you need to eat vegetables in abundance while you should have fruits at least two times a day.

Another food group that you need to eat daily is plant oils, such as olive, sesame, canola, soy, and vegetable oils. These are usually used when you are making your meals whether you include it as grease for your pan or you drizzle oil onto the food before serving. It is helpful to have a variety of oils in your home as you can choose a different oil to use whenever you make a dish. For example, if you make seafood pasta with vegetable oil the first time, you can switch to olive oil the next time. This will allow you to get a different taste and see which oil you like best with the dish.

Moving up the pyramid is fish and poultry. While some people consider this a daily food, the Mediterranean diet feels it is best to eat this no more than a few days of the week. The amount of daily servings on the food pyramid states 0 to 2, so you can eat these foods daily, but you also want to note how often you're eating them and what foods you're eating. For example, the Mediterranean diet supports seafood over poultry, so many people will eat more lobster, shrimp, and fish than chicken or turkey during the week.

Another weekly food group is dairy, which includes eggs, cheese, milk, and yogurt. You want to eat a little less of this group than you do seafood and poultry. You want to have a few servings throughout your week, but you don't need them on a daily basis.

Red meats and sweets you should eat sparingly. Foods included in this section include white bread, hamburger, steak, sausage, white rice, bacon, potatoes, and soda. Eating sparingly does not mean you should never touch it, though you can go this way if you want to and continue taking any supplements and vitamins you need to. It means that you should limit your servings to 0 to 2 a week. For instance, if you had a particularly bad day and are in need of a chocolate bar to make you feel better, go for it. As long as you have not eaten a lot of sweets that week, having a piece of candy on a weekly basis can benefit you mentally and emotionally. The trick is to have the self-discipline to say "no" to another candy bar that week.

At this point, it is important that you note that many people on the Mediterranean diet take vitamins and other supplements. This is because there are a lot of vitamins and minerals that poultry, dairy, and red meats hold, and your body needs these nutrients. Like any diet, if you are not careful with your meal plan and what foods you are putting into your body, you can find yourself lacking essential nutrients. If you need a calcium supplement because you only have dairy products a couple of times a week and your calcium is low, then you can easily purchase a calcium vitamin at a local store or pharmacy.

To break this down a bit, this is the daily allowance that you should generally follow. Of course, your health always comes first, so if you find yourself getting sick often or you feel that something is not right with your body, talk to your doctor as they can let you know if you are low on certain nutrients.

Olive oil is the oil you will use most often and can become a part of nearly every meal. It gives your food a great taste and you can also use it as a type of grease, so your food doesn't stick to the pan. When it comes to other foods that are included in your daily allowance, you can have up to three servings of dairy products and fruit. You should have about six servings of vegetables and up to eight servings of brown rice, whole grain bread, and other non-refined products.

When it comes to your weekly allowance, you should limit your servings of potatoes, sweets, and eggs to three. You can have up to four servings of olives, poultry, nuts, and legumes. You should have no more than six servings of fish and other seafood. While you will eat olive oil often, you should watch how many tablespoons and limit it to 14 for a weekly total.

The item on most people's grocery list that you should have the least of is red meat, which is about four servings a month or one serving a week. This means that any pork, veal, or beef needs to take a back seat to other meats. You do not need to avoid red meat, though some people on the Mediterranean diet do, but limiting it is important. If you need to, remember to divide your servings up throughout the week so you can help calm any cravings that you feel are becoming uncontrollable.

Food Lists

Now that you have an idea of the Mediterranean food pyramid, it is time to look at what foods you can place on your plate and whether there are foods you should avoid entirely. Surprisingly, the food pyramid does not have any foods that you absolutely have to avoid, which means the avoidance list is completely optional. It is there for you, so you know to limit these foods as much as possible. Of course, you can follow the path of many other dieters and decide to follow the avoidance list just so that your body will be completely free from these foods.

Mediterranean foods that you can put on your daily list include:

- Olives
- Olive oil
- Avocado oil
- Non-starchy vegetables
- Starchy vegetables
- Fruit
- Anything that is whole-grain
- Oatmeal
- Balsamic vinegar
- Pesto
- Tomato sauce but without sugar
- Water
- Tea
- Coffee
- Herbs
- Spices
- Garlic
- Tofu
- Seitan
- Beans
- Tempeh
- Chickpeas
- Lentils

Mediterranean foods that you can eat often, but usually not every day:

- Fish
- Pistachios
- Cashews
- Eggs
- Seafood
- Walnuts
- Almonds
- Hazelnuts
- Chicken
- Canola oil
- All-bran cereals
- Pasta that is not whole-grain, but you should generally try to eat whole-grain
- Plain ricotta
- Cottage cheese
- Any type of cheese
- Plain Greek yogurt
- Milk
- Adding a small amount of sugar to tea, coffee, or any other foods
- Honey
- Red wine or other types of alcohol
- Salting food to taste

There are foods that you should eat sparingly or avoid if you choose. One characteristic of the Mediterranean diet is it doesn't force you to stay away from any foods like other diets do. However, this diet focuses on healthy fats and carbohydrates, which are not available in all foods. There are more unhealthy fats and carbohydrates in these selected foods:

- Frozen pancakes
- Frozen waffles
- Fruit juice
- Soda
- Sweetened coffee or tea
- Sweetened nut butters
- Sweetened trail mixes
- Ice cream
- Sugar-sweetened cereals
- White sugar
- Nuts with sugar
- Snack foods, such as crackers
- Trans fats
- Red meat
- Butter and margarine
- Bacon
- Processed meats, such as hot dogs and chicken nuggets
- Ketchup
- BBQ sauce
- Teriyaki sauce
- Processed cheese, such as American
- Sweetened yogurt

Cleaning out Your Cupboards

When you start the Mediterranean diet, it's hard to open your cupboards, pantry, freezer, and fridge and note what foods you need to eat sparingly or avoid. For most people, this is especially true when it comes to their favorite snacks, such as chips. While you can decide to leave these foods in your home and eat them rarely, it is usually best to start the diet with the foods you shouldn't eat often out of your home. This will give you a better success rate as you will not feel tempted to have a handful of chips every day or grab that steak instead of the fish.

First, you want to go through your cupboards, fridge, and pantry and clean out all the old snacks, food, and stale food. This story happens to nearly everyone—you are busy and with other people rummaging through your cupboards for snacks throughout the day, it is hard to notice what cereal boxes are low, what cereal is stale, and what foods have hit their expiration date. Taking care of these items will quickly start cutting down on the sugary and unhealthy food as you start the Mediterranean diet.

Second, you want to think about the other people in your household. If you're the only person on the Mediterranean diet, you will continue to have foods and other snacks available for your family that you shouldn't eat. The best tip for this situation is to do your best to keep the "bad" foods out of sight and out of mind. For example, your significant other can hide the foods from you but know where they are for the rest of the family. If this isn't an option, you can place the foods in an area where you do not see them daily and where your children can reach them. This way, when your child asks for a fruit snack, you can tell them where it is, but you don't need to bring a package to them. Furthermore, even if you buy the food and you know where it is, you are less likely to eat it if you need to take a few more steps, open the door, and take out the item.

Third, you can always find people to take food that does not follow the Mediterranean diet. For instance, you might have a friend with a few little children who would love the bad snacks, or you have friends that aren't on a diet and will take the food out of your cupboards. If you are getting rid of unopened, non-perishable packaged foods, you can take them to a local food pantry. Of course, you will want to check the expiration dates so you don't bring old items to the food pantry.

Finally, you want to stop and think before you add more food to your cupboards. When you're grocery shopping, make a list of the ingredients you need and ignore the ones you don't. It's not easy to walk away from the unhealthy foods that you love, but if you make it a point to write out a grocery list, stick to it, and tell yourself "no" and walk away when the wrong foods become tempting, then following your meal plan and staying on the path will become easier.

Notes:

Chapter 3: Your Meal Planning Guide

Meal prepping are two words that ring in the ears of every busy person. You know that planning your meals will help you, but you don't know where to begin. You think it's as simple as writing down which meals you want to eat that week, making them when you have free time, storing them in the fridge or freezer, and then warming them up when you get home. However, when you go down this route, you quickly learn that it's not as easy as you originally thought. In fact, there is a lot of planning, guidelines, and organizing that you need to follow to ensure you plan your meals on a weekly basis.

When it comes to meal planning, the foundation is based on determination and self-discipline. There are other ingredients that you will need, but without these two factors, you won't find yourself sticking to your meal planning routine. You need to have the determination to succeed with planning and the self-discipline to tell yourself to stop reading your book or turn off the television and get into the kitchen to prepare your meals for the week. When you have a busy life, these factors are difficult because you value your time to relax and unwind. You decide to push aside making the meals during the weekend not because you're lazy, which is what you might think, but because your body is tired, and you need to rest.

One way to help you find your drive to prepare meals when you need to be to think about how much easier your evenings are when you have prepared meals. This is true whether you live alone or have a family to take care of.

Getting Started on Your Meal Plan

However, before you find your drive to succeed with meal planning, you need to get started on your plan. This first step is difficult for most people, so don't worry if you're thinking, "How do I do that?"

Step one when it comes to getting started is to not feel overwhelmed. It's easy to feel this way because meal planning is a lot of work, especially when you're not sure what you're doing. Take a deep breath and tell yourself, "I got this" because you do. Don't think of the little details when it comes to planning your weekly meals and don't focus too much on the details. The trick to meal planning is you take it one day at the time, one meal at a time, and it becomes a much easier task.

Step two focuses on picking a day. Don't wait till you wake up one morning and think to yourself, "I will start planning my meals today." You're more likely to put it off when it comes down to writing down your meals and preparing your grocery list because you're not mentally prepared to start meal planning. You need to get into the correct mindset. One way to do this is by imagining your future. Think of how easy your days will become once you start planning your daily meals. If you need help when it comes to the mindset, keep a journal that allows you to focus on what your goals are and how you're meeting them. For example, if you're following the Mediterranean diet because you want to eat healthier, discuss the foods you're eating.

Another point when it comes to picking a day is to settle on a day to work on your meal planning and prepping. Some people will start on Saturdays and go into Sunday. For example, they will write down what meals they plan to eat for the following week and prepare their grocery shopping list on Saturday. The next day, they will go grocery shopping, come home, and immediately start preparing the meals by chopping the vegetables, fruit, and making the meals they can. Other people make their meal plan and gather their list on Wednesday and then go shopping on Saturday night and start making their meals on Sunday. You need to find a flow that works for you, and it might take a couple of weeks, but once you find it you will feel it.

Step three looks at picking the meals for the week. To do this, you can write down your favorite meals first and then fill in the other meals by looking through a cookbook. This might be a little more challenging when you first start the Mediterranean diet, but once you start trying it out, you'll find that everything is a lot easier by week two or three.

Another point to consider when starting is to focus on some meals that you know well. Even if all your meals are not Mediterranean style the first week or two, this is fine. You can incorporate Mediterranean meals slowly into your weeks. When you focus on meals that you know, especially during your first week, you'll feel more confident about the process.

Step four focuses on making your grocery list. You can start your list when you start looking through your cupboards to see what you have available and what ingredients you will need to purchase. When making your list, one great tip is to think of the grocery store you will shop at and write down your items in order. This means if your grocery store starts with fruits and vegetables, you will write these items down first. Then, you go on to the next section of the store. Following this tip helps you stick to your list because you're following it in order and you don't need to stop and check to see if you need something from the aisle or not, you easily know because it is next on your list.

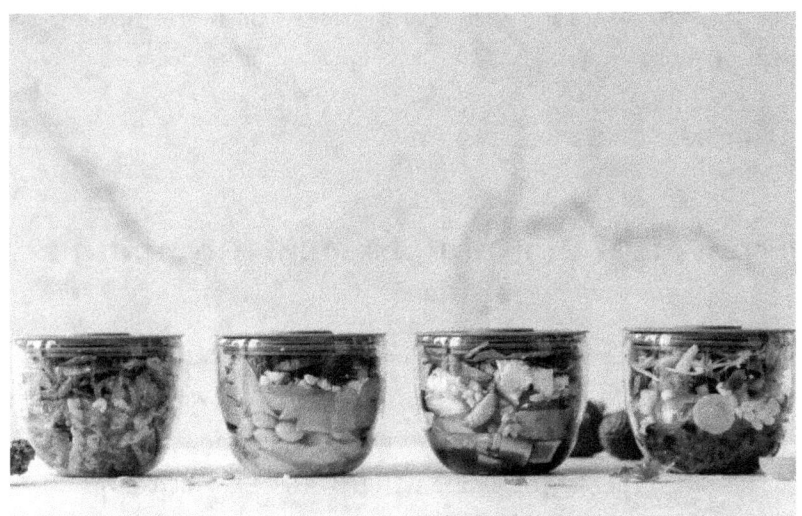

Step five looks at making sure you have the right containers. You don't want to store everything in baggies because they are not tightly sealed, and air can leak through. The best containers are airtight and can divide into sections. There are recipes, such as casseroles, that you can make and store all of it in one container. Then, there are other meals where you'll want to keep ingredients separated until the night you eat the meal.

Part of step five is learning how to enjoy your leftovers. This is not easy for everyone because some people do not like food after the second day. When you're meal planning, you will plan to make so many meals and eat them for a day or two. For example, you will make mushroom lasagna Sunday night and divide the leftovers into containers for your work lunches. You'll also make meals during the weekend that you'll pack away after they cool and save for later in the week, such as Thursday night. The trick is to make sure that you can store the meal for a few days without it going bad.

From Meal Planning to Meal Prepping

Now that you've learned a bit about how to start your meal-planning guide, you need to think about how you will plan and prepare your meals. When you're planning, you're writing down what meals you will eat for the week, such as what is compiled in Chapters 5 through 8. When you're prepping your meals, you're not only planning them but you're starting to make them and will store them in containers to eat throughout the week.

You need to look at your calendar to see what day(s) work best to prepare your meals, whether you want to do it immediately after your weekly grocery shopping trip, and how many nights you want to make dinner at home. One of the best benefits of the Mediterranean diet is you don't always need to eat at home. You can go to nearly every restaurant and find something suitable to eat that follows the diet. You might receive more unhealthy food, depending on what you order, but if you choose seafood, whole-wheat, whole-grain, vegetables, and fruits you are sticking with the diet.

Another factor you need to consider is what foods you can prepare and what ones you need to wait to make. For example, you probably do not want to bake your fish and then put it in the fridge for a couple of days. Instead, get your fish ready by washing it and taking any bones out if you choose and then put the fish in an airtight container until fish night. You also won't want to make your salads ahead of time, but you might consider making your lasagna a couple of days before lasagna night.

Chopping your fruits, vegetables, and even grilling chicken to cut up and freeze for later in the week is a great start to your meal prepping. These steps will also decrease the amount of time you spend in the kitchen after a busy weekday.

Organizing Your Meal Plan

One of the biggest reasons people walk away from meal planning is because they become overwhelmed by planning and organizing their meals. Planning is very basic, you go through recipes and write down what you want to eat and when. The trick is to stick within your calorie limit and watch what foods you eat in a day. For example, on the Mediterranean diet, you won't want to make two meals with chicken or red meat in one day. However, you will want to make two meals that focus on vegetables, at least one that has fruit, add some seafood at least 5 times a week, and include nuts, seeds, oils, herbs, and cheese.

Don't think of meal planning as a huge binder with dozens of recipes that are falling out everywhere. If this is your style and helps you feel organized, you can use this method. But, most people like to keep their meal planning organization on their computer. For instance, they will have a spreadsheet of all the meals they make with nutritional information and then divide and conquer with the meal list every week. You could have Monday, Wednesday, Friday, and Sunday as your seafood nights and reserve Saturday night for chicken or red meat, which you might alternate. You could decide that you will have a big breakfast on Sunday mornings where you make sausage and use this as your red meat day during the week. These choices are completely up to you. It's easier than people think to create a meal plan on the Mediterranean diet because you mainly focus on foods you're used to, but eat more vegetables, fruits, seafood, oils, and whole-grains.

One tip to help you stay organized with meal planning is to keep your recipes organized. You can do this by copying them into a spreadsheet or through a recipe box. It might become easier to have all your recipes in one area than several recipe books lying all over your table during meal planning night.

Another tip is to not be shy about trying new recipes. One reason so many recipes are included in this book is that it's important to keep your mind open and try a new dish at least once a week. Not only does this expand your meal planning list, but it also keeps your family interested in the new weekly dish.

Another tip to help you with organization is realizing that you don't need to make all the meals from scratch. If you find a box of suddenly salad with whole-wheat macaroni and vegetables, check out the nutritional information. If it fits in your diet, go ahead and try it out.

The biggest tip to follow when organizing your meal plan is don't pay attention to anyone else's organizational methods. You need to find your method and then stick with it. For example, you might write down your meal plans on a piece of paper and hang it on the fridge. You might make your plan on your laptop through Microsoft Excel. No matter what method you find, you need to be comfortable with it and it needs to work with you and no one else. Also, don't feel bad when you have a night that you're simply too tired to cook and decide to pick up a salad and chicken from the grocery store. These nights happen from time to time.

Sticking to Your Budget

One of the hardest parts of grocery shopping, whether you're on a diet or not, is sticking to your budget. You know it—food is expensive, and its prices seem to climb faster than your income. Many people state that one reason they don't stick to diets is that they can't afford some of the food. Fortunately, this is not the problem on the Mediterranean diet because there are very few foods that you can't eat. The most expensive foods are some types of seafood.

When it comes to tips on sticking to your budget, one of the first you'll receive is to create a meal plan. You can now say "check" because you're well on your way to completing this step.

Another factor is one that was already briefly discussed, and this is purchasing foods when they are on sale. Go through the sales in the newspaper and advertisements. Go online to check your local grocery store's website and see what type of sales they have for the week. If you know that you'll make a meal with a certain ingredient in the future or you see an ingredient you use often, even if it isn't in your meal plan for the week, go ahead and stock up. You will save some money down the road when you follow this method.

Meat is one of the most expensive parts of grocery shopping, especially on the Mediterranean diet. Decide to eat a little less seafood on weeks that you know money is tighter than normal, such as when rent is due. Instead, focus more on dairy, beans, and canned fish like tuna.

Another tip is to get a little creative with your meals. You can eat whole-grains on the Mediterranean diet and these ingredients are often bought in bulk. Buy that bigger bag of whole-grain pasta and rice and use it for a couple of weeks. You might need a break from rice after 2 to 3 weeks, but this will allow you to focus on different meals during that week.

Making a little more than what you need for one meal to ensure you have leftovers is another great way to save a little money. This will allow you to take the leftovers to work for lunch or have them the following night. You can also keep most meals in airtight containers in the freezer for a couple of months. Doing this with leftovers can help you with your meal planning down the road.

Finally, when you're preparing your meals and grocery list, think of what your family eats. If you know they aren't big fans of rice, don't make a lot of meals with rice. Focus more on pasta and vegetables that they will eat as this will decrease the amount of leftovers, and possibly waste, that you have to deal with.

Notes:

Chapter 4: Your Grocery Shopping Guide

If you are like most people, you look for deals when you go grocery shopping. You have a budget and you need to stick to it. One myth of the Mediterranean diet is that you cannot buy healthy food on a budget. While some food is a bit more on the expensive side, the majority of Mediterranean friendly food will fit your budget. The key to grocery shopping is to follow a few tips, such as making a list of items you need before you go, sticking to the list while shopping, and not shopping on an empty stomach.

Before You Go Shopping

The first step is to know where you will shop. You might already have a favorite grocery store and know where everything is, or you might shop at several different stores. The best tip is to find the cheapest grocery store that has the items you need for the Mediterranean diet and make this your primary store. You might also decide to stop at superstores, such as Walmart, so you can get everything you need in one trip.

One factor to consider when you start looking at which store is best is coupons, store specials, and a large selection of fruits, vegetables, seafood, and other essentials for the diet. There are some stores that will have smaller selections when it comes to fresh fruits and vegetables because they do take up a lot of room.

Another factor to consider is the quality of the food. Take a careful look at how they keep their fresh produce and how it looks before you buy it. For example, do they water down some of their fruits and vegetables to help keep them fresh? Is the area cool enough? Does it look like it's healthy or are there several spots that show the produce is about to rot? Think of the smell when you walk by the produce and notice if it smells fresh or if there is a smell in there that isn't something you want to bring home.

Once you have chosen your store, you can move on to the second step which is to get to know your store. Walk around and understand their layout. Most grocery stores have a similar layout, but some stores like to change things up. Make notes of the layout or take pictures so you know the order and can write down the items you need in order.

Tips to Give You the Best Shopping Experience

One tip is to make sure you have a tally or a calculator with you. This will help you stay within your budget as you can calculate how much your items will cost as you place them in the cart. You can also find the cheapest items if the store carries more than one brand of a certain ingredient.

A second tip is to bring your receipt home and keep it in a spreadsheet. This will help you manage your budget as you will start to get an idea of how much you spend on a weekly basis, what items you use the most, and if you spend more money during certain times of the month or year. You can also use this to plan your grocery budget a bit more accurately. For example, if you notice that the second week of the month is the time you usually spend the most, you'll know to prepare for this.

A third tip is that you can work on your shopping list throughout the week. If you're making dinner and you notice that you're running low on tuna, write it down on your list. This will help you save time when it comes to your meal planning day.

Fourth, comparison shopping can be incredibly beneficial to your budget. You can do this at the store when it comes to similar items or with coupons. Sometimes, you'll notice that some stores have better deals than others. If you come across this, take a closer look at the store with the better deals and see if they have all the items that you need. Even if you're only saving a couple of dollars every week, this can go a long way in a year.

Fifth, check your list before you check out at the store. It's easy to miss an item, especially when you're short on time. This will help you ensure you have everything that you need so you don't have to run back to the store later in the week.

Finally, you want to always ensure that you have a list. Even if you're running to the store for a couple of items because you decided to make a surprise meal or you find a recipe you really want to try out for your evening meal, you need to write down everything on your list. It doesn't matter if it is a couple of items or several, making a grocery list will help you stay on target and keep track of your budget.

Creating Your Grocery List

You can go about creating your list and meal planning in multiple ways, a few of which we'll list here, or you can come up with a different system that works for you. For example, you might look at the coupons before you write out your meal list, so you have an easier time staying in your budget. You might also have a meal planning system that you follow so it's easier to pick meals for the week, and you can follow this when it comes to creating your grocery list. No matter what system you follow, it needs to be the right system for you.

Organization is a key factor when it comes to making your grocery list. To create an organized list, you can follow these steps.

First, always create your meal plan. You already read about this, but it is incredibly important when you're creating your grocery list and is the first step in your process. You have to know what meals you're making so you know exactly what items you need.

Second, go through your cabinets, freezer, fridge, and pantry. Write down the items that you need and do not have or write down the items that you have. This will help guide you when it comes to creating your grocery list. Don't forget about the amount of the ingredients that you have. For instance, if you need almond flour for a few meals and notice you're running low, you need to put it on your list.

Third, you will organize your list by thinking about the store you chose. You might not get the items in the correct order all of the time, but you will be close. You can do this by separating your list into different sections. For example, if vegetables are first when it comes to the store, write down what vegetables you need at the top of the list. Then go on to fruits, canned goods, frozen foods, and so on. You can create your own template on Microsoft Word to make creating your grocery list easier or you can find a template online and download it.

Fourth, double-check your list before you leave your house. Make sure that the items you wrote down are not in your home. Match the items to the ingredients on your recipes and make sure they are in your pantry if you don't have them on the list or aren't in your pantry if you do. For example, if you have almond butter on the recipe and it's on your list, look at where you keep that item to make sure you need to buy it this week.

Chapter 5 has a week one meal plan for the Mediterranean diet. You can practice writing out your first grocery list by looking at the meals written down and the ingredients you have in your home. If the meal is something you've never made before, check to see if the recipe is included in Chapter 9. Of course, you can always find a suitable recipe online through a quick Google search. However, most of the meals are easy and you can add any herbs and oils that you want. You can even switch out vegetables and fruits to include your favorite ones. For example, the first meal is "Whole grain toast with one egg and a side of fruit. You can pan-fry your egg, scramble, or boil it. Coffee or tea is a great choice for a beverage." Look in your kitchen and see if you have eggs, whole grain bread, fruit, coffee, or tea. If you have all of these items in your home, move on to the next meal. If you notice you are low on eggs or bread, write these items on your list.

Notes:

Chapter 5: Week One Meal Plan

When your first week on the diet comes, one of the first factors you should expect is that this week will feel the hardest. How well you follow the diet and ensure you're getting all the nutrients you need will affect how strongly you feel any cravings. If you have incredibly strong cravings that are hard to control, look at your meal plan and compare it to the food you are craving. Look to see if you're missing anything in your diet. Fortunately, this is rare and usually happens when you stick to a few foods during the week. For instance, if you only eat fruits twice a week or you decide to skip placing seafood on your diet during the week.

This meal plan is only a guide. You don't have to follow it food by food, but you should watch what foods you change. For example, if you don't like blueberries, you'll want to replace them with another fruit. This will help you keep your meal plan balanced and further guide you when you begin making your own meal plans.

Just like this chapter will have a few recipes, the following three chapters will follow the same format. I will include recipes for items that are not commonly known in chapter 9. For example, it is easy to combine Greek yogurt with blueberries for your breakfast, but you might not know how to make mushroom lasagna for your dinner. Thus, I will include that recipe here for your convenience.

Monday

Breakfast: Whole grain toast with one egg and a side of fruit. You can pan-fry your egg, scramble, or boil it. Coffee or tea is a great choice for a beverage.

Lunch: A tossed salad with vegetables, white beans, and olives. For more protein in your diet, you can also bake a small piece of chicken. You want to ensure you have protein in your lunch if you skipped the egg for breakfast. For lunch, it's best to have a glass of water. To give it a little more flavor, you can add lemon or lime.

Dinner: Boiled artichoke, drizzled with olive oil and seasoned with a dash of salt and garlic powder. Steam two cups of spinach and sprinkle with your favorite herbs, lime juice, or lemon juice. You can relax with a glass of wine, water, or have another nice cup of tea. If you have not had any dairy, a glass of skim milk is suitable.

Snack ideas: If you find yourself hungry during the day, grabbing a few baby carrots is a great morning snack because you had fruit for breakfast. For an afternoon snack, you can eat a cup of Greek yogurt or have an apple with almond butter.

Tuesday

Breakfast: Using a wide-mouth jar or a bowl, fill half of it with Greek yogurt. Take 1 cup of raspberries, blueberries, or blackberries and add to the top. For a little crunch, you can also add about ¼ cup of granola. Have a cup of coffee, tea, or flavored water.

Lunch: Tuna salad with a drizzle of olive oil. You can add your favorite piece of fruit as a side and have a glass of water with lemon.

Dinner: Salad with Brussels sprouts and chickpeas and leftover tuna salad that you can make into a sandwich on whole-grain bread. Your salad will taste even better with a glass of water or red wine.

Snack ideas: Grab a piece of whole-grain bread or flatbread and 2 tablespoons of hummus. Mix a little olive oil, salt, and pepper into your hummus to give it a different taste and spread over the bread. You can also include your favorite seasonings or a different type of oil.

This salad can sit in the fridge for up to four days. It's a great salad to make during the weekend and take to work for the first few days of the week!

Wednesday

Breakfast: Oatmeal topped with a few raisins and a small glass of milk. Some people feel the milk tastes better when it has been warmed up a bit.

Lunch: Leftover tuna salad from the night before with a piece of fruit or a side of vegetables. A glass of water with a little lemon or lime for added taste.

Dinner: Whole-grain sandwich with a side of mixed vegetables. A glass of red or white wine.

Snack ideas: Celery with a little almond butter or a piece of fruit.

Thursday

Breakfast: One egg omelet with a mix of vegetables. Adding a bowl of fruit can help keep your energy up until lunch. You could also have a glass of freshly squeezed orange juice.

Lunch: Whole grain sandwich with a side of vegetables. A glass of water with lemon or lime.

Dinner: Vegetarian lasagna roll-ups.

Snack ideas: ¼ cup of almonds, cashews, or sunflower seeds. You can also create your own mix and add a little dried fruit.

Friday

Breakfast: 1 cup of whole-grain oats mixed with a little honey and cinnamon. You can also add some blueberries or raspberries instead of honey or cinnamon. To give your oats more crunch and taste, you can also add about a ½ cup of sliced almonds.

Lunch: Leftover lasagna from the previous evening.

Dinner: Boil about 1 cup of white beans and mix with garlic, basil, Italian seasoning, avocado oil, or any other herbs and oils. Measure 1 cup of arugula with a little cheese and olive oil as a dressing.

Snack ideas: Frozen blueberry yogurt or baby carrots.

Saturday

Breakfast: Scrambled eggs, no more than two eggs, with a mix of vegetables, such as tomatoes and onions. A glass of freshly squeezed juice or a cup of coffee.

Lunch: Whole-grain tuna sandwich with a cup of fruit. A glass of water that you can add lemon too for extra flavor.

Dinner: Grilled chicken with a side of steamed or roasted vegetables. You can also have a little treat for the week and grab a can of soda. Of course, a glass of wine also works well with your meal.

Snack ideas: Dried fruit with a few cashews or a handful of pistachios.

Sunday

Breakfast: One or two slices of whole-grain toast with almond butter and a side of fruit. A cup of coffee is suitable to help you get started on your relaxing day.

Lunch: Vegetable soup with whole-grain crackers.

Dinner: Steam two cups of kale and mix with tomatoes, cheese, lemon juice, and cucumbers. Grill a fish fillet or have a bowl of tuna and a glass of red wine.

Snack ideas: Roasted chickpeas or hummus with veggies.

Notes:

Chapter 6: Week Two Meal Plan

Monday

Breakfast: Scrambled eggs with spinach, tomatoes, and a cup of coffee.

Lunch: Arugula salad with lemon, parmesan cheese, and olive oil. Wash your salad down with a glass of water.

Dinner: Baked salmon that is garnished with dill and a side of fruit. You can have a glass of wine or flavored water.

Snack ideas: A handful of almonds or a strawberry smoothie.

Tuesday

Breakfast: Lettuce, tomato, and avocado on whole-grain toast. A cup of coffee or freshly squeezed juice is best for a drink.

Lunch: Cucumber salad with chopped onions. To make a little dressing, mix water, white vinegar, and salt to taste. Include a glass of water with this meal.

Dinner: Baked chicken with a mix of vegetables and a glass of water or wine.

Snack ideas: Baby carrots, a banana, or sliced apples.

Wednesday

Breakfast: Omelet with chopped broccoli and cheese. A cup of coffee or freshly squeezed orange juice.

Lunch: A salad with beans, olives, shredded carrots, and cheese. You can also make a small piece of chicken to chop into the salad or have on the side. A glass of milk or water to drink.

Dinner: Mediterranean pizza on a whole-wheat crust with a glass of water or milk, depending on which one you did not have for lunch.

Snack ideas: Mix of fruit or apples with almond butter.

Thursday

Breakfast: Scrambled eggs and vegetable mix with a cup of coffee.

Lunch: Tuna on whole-grain bread and a side of fruit or leftover pizza from the previous night. A glass of milk or water is perfect for this meal.

Dinner: Hamburgers with french fries and a glass of milk.

Snack ideas: Yogurt and a peach.

Friday

Breakfast: Whole-grain oats with dates and cinnamon. You can also add a side of fruit or include the fruit in your oats. A glass of freshly squeezed orange juice is a perfect companion for this heart-healthy breakfast.

Lunch: Cucumber salad or a regular salad with your favorite toppings. A glass of water with a slice of lime.

Dinner: Fish cooked in olive oil with your favorite seasonings and a side of your favorite vegetables. A glass of water or red wine.

Snack ideas: A piece of fruit, a handful of nuts, or a couple of cheese slices with other veggies.

Saturday

Breakfast: Bulgur fruit breakfast bowl and a cup of tea or coffee.

Lunch: Whole-grain sandwich with a slice of cheese and a side of vegetables. A glass of milk or water.

Dinner: Oven-roasted mixed vegetables with a side of whole-wheat or whole-grain flatbread. You can also have a small piece of chicken or turkey. A glass of wine or water.

Snack ideas: Baby carrots or a handful of your favorite nuts.

Sunday

Breakfast: 1 cup of Greek yogurt with a few raspberries and a cup of coffee or freshly squeezed juice.

Lunch: 2 cups of mixed salad greens topped with cherry tomatoes, cheese, shredded carrots, or cucumbers. A glass of water with lemon.

Dinner: Grilled lamb with a side of grilled vegetables and a glass of milk or wine.

Snack ideas: Dried fruit, banana, or a ½ cup of nuts.

Notes:

Chapter 7: Week Three Meal Plan

Monday

Breakfast: Poached egg on whole-wheat toast with a side of fruit. A cup of coffee, freshly squeezed juice, or milk is a perfect drink.

Lunch: Soup with ham and peas and a glass of water with lemon.

Dinner: Bass or another type of fish with dill relish. A glass of wine, milk (if you haven't had too much dairy) or water to drink.

Snack ideas: Frozen yogurt or baked apples.

Tuesday

Breakfast: Two slices of whole-wheat avocado toast and a cup of coffee.

Lunch: Salad with your favorite vegetables and olive oil as dressing. You can also add any herbs or another type of oil for more flavor. Serve with a glass of water and a slice of lemon.

Dinner: Garlic and cajun shrimp bowl with noodles and a glass of red wine.

Snack ideas: Bowl of mixed fruit.

Wednesday

Breakfast: Whole grain toast with one egg and a side of fruit. You can poach or pan-fry your egg. A cup of coffee or a glass of freshly squeezed orange juice.

Lunch: Tomato and basil soup with a glass of milk. You can also have a grilled cheese sandwich on whole-grain bread.

Dinner: Grilled salmon with a side salad topped with your favorite vegetables. A glass of red wine, water, or a glass of milk.

Snack ideas: Strawberry popsicle or a bowl of fruit.

Thursday

Breakfast: Greek yogurt topped with fruit and a cup of coffee.

Lunch: Steam mixed vegetables and have a slice of whole-grain bread with almond butter. You could also make a sandwich with a little tuna and cheese. Include a glass of water or milk to drink.

Dinner: Grilled calamari with berries and a glass of red wine.

Snack ideas: Steamed vegetables or a ¼ cup of nuts.

Friday

Breakfast: Whole-grain oatmeal with cinnamon and topped with berries. A cup of coffee or freshly squeezed orange juice to drink.

Lunch: Hard-boiled egg crushed on a slice of whole-grain toast and a side of vegetables. A glass of water with a slice of lemon.

Dinner: Don't forget about a date night or family night in your favorite restaurant! Most places have plenty of Mediterranean type options, such as grilled fish and a salad or a side of steamed vegetables. Don't think that just because you eat the Mediterranean way you can't enjoy a night at your favorite neighborhood spot.

Snack ideas: A handful of almonds or baby carrots. Another option is celery or apples with almond butter.

Saturday

Breakfast: Scrambled eggs with a bowl of fruit. For a drink, a cup of coffee or freshly squeezed orange juice.

Lunch: Steam two cups of spinach and sprinkle with your favorite herbs, lime juice, or lemon juice. Include some boiled artichoke hearts drizzled with olive oil and seasoned with a dash of garlic powder and sea salt. Have a glass of milk or water to drink.

Dinner: Grilled pork chop with steamed vegetables or a baked potato. Enjoy this rare and special meal with a glass of red wine.

Snack ideas: Chunky monkey trail mix.

Sunday

Breakfast: One egg with a slice of avocado toast. Freshly squeezed orange juice or a cup of coffee to drink.

Lunch: Whole-grain tuna sandwich with a slice of cheese and a cup of fruit. A glass of water that you can add lemon too for more flavor.

Dinner: Spinach and beans salad with a Mediterranean taste and a glass of white wine.

Snack ideas: Chunky monkey trail mix, pineapple chunks or rings, or orange slices.

Notes:

Chapter 8: Week Four Meal Plan

Monday

Breakfast: Scrambled eggs with spinach, tomatoes, and a cup of coffee.

Lunch: Whole-grain sandwich with a slice of cheese and a side of vegetables. A glass of water with lemon or lime.

Dinner: Boiled artichoke with avocado or olive oil and a little paprika or garlic powder. Two cups of steamed vegetables with lime juice sprinkled on top. A glass of wine for a relaxing drink.

Snack ideas: Mix of fruit or apples with almond butter.

Tuesday

Breakfast: Whole grain toast with one egg, a side of fruit, and tea or coffee.

Lunch: Whole grain sandwich with a side of vegetables. A glass of water with lemon is perfect for a drink.

Dinner: Oven-roasted mixed vegetables with a side of whole-grain flatbread and a small piece of chicken. A glass of wine or water.

Snack ideas: Baby carrots or an apple with almond butter.

Wednesday

Breakfast: An omelet with a little cheese and a bowl of fruit. A glass of freshly squeezed orange juice, tea, or coffee.

Lunch: A tossed salad with vegetables, white beans, and olives. One of the best lunch drinks is a glass of water with a slice of lemon.

Dinner: Vegetable soup with whole-grain crackers and a glass of milk.

Snack ideas: Apples, banana, or a bowl of mixed berries.

Thursday

Breakfast: One or two slices of whole-grain toast with almond butter, a side of fruit, and a cup of tea.

Lunch: 2 cups of mixed salad greens topped with cherry tomatoes, cheese, shredded carrots, or cucumbers. A glass of water or milk to drink.

Dinner: Mediterranean pizza on whole-wheat crust with a glass of water or wine.

Snack ideas: Roasted chickpeas or hummus with veggies.

Friday

Breakfast: Bulgur fruit breakfast bowl and a cup of tea or coffee.

Lunch: Tuna salad sandwich on whole-grain bread or flatbread and a side of veggies or fruit. A glass of water with lemon to drink.

Dinner: Steam two cups of kale and mix with tomatoes, cheese, lemon juice, cucumbers, and a bowl of tuna. A glass of wine or milk is a great drink.

Snack ideas: Yogurt or your favorite vegetable.

Saturday

Breakfast: Greek quinoa breakfast bowl with a cup of coffee.

Lunch: A tossed salad with vegetables on top. Use your favorite vinaigrette to add a little flavor. For a drink, use a glass of water with a side of lemon.

Dinner: Mediterranean pizza with whole-wheat crust. You can even give yourself a little treat by having a can of soda.

Snack ideas: A bowl of berries or apples and almond butter.

Sunday

Breakfast: Omelet with chopped broccoli and cheese. A cup of coffee or freshly squeezed orange juice.

Lunch: Salad with Brussels sprouts and chickpeas. Your salad will taste even better with a glass of water and a slice of lemon or lime.

Dinner: Grilled fish with a side of fruit and a glass of red wine.

Snack ideas: A handful of almonds or another type of nut. You can even create a little mix with a few raisins.

A professional tip when it comes to meal planning is that you want to create a guideline that you follow every week. For example, if you want to stick to a 1,800 calorie diet, then you should write how many calories are in each dish and add them together to ensure that you are under your calorie intake. If you want to focus more on healthy fat content than carbs, you will note this with your dishes. An example of a meal prep guideline is below.

Breakfast: I will grab something that is easy and quick or premake a meal the night before. The meal should be fine when it comes to sitting in the fridge for at least five days. I will focus on freshly squeezed juice or have a cup of coffee to drink.

Lunch: Prepare meals that focus on vegetables and I can easily package and take to work with me. Leftovers from the night before are always a great idea. I will try to stick to a glass of water to drink.

Dinner: Meals should focus on healthy fats, protein, and the main food groups I need on the Mediterranean diet. If I haven't had enough fruits or vegetables, I can add these to the meal. To drink, I can have a small glass of red wine, water, or a glass of milk. The meal needs to feed a family of 3.

Snack: Focus on light snacks that will cure the appetite. I'll either have something I can quickly put into a baggie or something I can pack with my lunch.

Nutritional goals: To eat a well-balanced meal every day and make sure I eat the food groups I need to. For my goal, eating healthy is more important than counting calories.

Notes:

Chapter 9: Mediterranean Recipes

Breakfast

Greek Quinoa Breakfast Bowl

Time: 30 minutes

Servings: 6

Ingredients:

- 12 eggs
- 1 teaspoon onion powder
- ½ teaspoon salt
- 1 teaspoon olive oil
- 1 pint halved cherry tomatoes
- 2 cups cooked quinoa
- ¼ cup Greek yogurt, plain
- 1 teaspoon garlic powder
- ½ teaspoon black pepper
- 5 ounces of baby spinach
- 1 cup feta cheese

Directions:

1. Add the eggs into a bowl and whisk thoroughly.
2. Combine the onion powder, garlic powder, Greek yogurt, pepper, and salt. Mix well.
3. Turn a stove burner to medium heat and place a large skillet on the burner. Allow it to heat up for about a minute.

4. Pour in the olive oil and toss in the spinach. Cook for 3 to 4 minutes or until the spinach becomes wilted.
5. Combine the cherry tomatoes into the skillet. Cook for another 3 minutes while stirring occasionally.
6. Add the eggs into the skillet and cook until they are set, which should take between 6 to 8 minutes. Stir the eggs often as you want them to look scrambled.
7. Add in the feta and quinoa. Continue to cook the mixture until all the ingredients are cooked thoroughly. You can store this breakfast for four days in the fridge.

Nutritional facts: calories: 252, fats: 16 grams, carbohydrates: 18 grams, protein: 10 grams.

Bulgur Fruit Breakfast Bowl

Time: 15 minutes

Servings: 6

Ingredients:

- 2 cups 2% milk
- ½ teaspoon ground cinnamon
- 1 ½ cups bulgur
- ½ cup almonds, chopped
- ½ cup mint, chopped (fresh is preferred)
- 8 dried and chopped figs
- 1 cup water
- 2 cups frozen sweet cherries - you can also substitute in blueberries or blackberries

Directions:

1. Turn your stovetop to medium heat and combine the bulger, water, milk, and cinnamon. Lightly stir as the ingredients come to a boil.
2. Cover your mixture and turn the stove range temperature down to medium-low heat. Let the mixture simmer for 8 to 11 minutes. It is done simmering when about half of the liquid has been absorbed
3. Without removing the pan, turn off the rangetop heat and add the frozen cherries, almonds, and figs. Lightly stir and then cover for one minute so the cherries can thaw, and the mixture can combine.
4. Remove the cover and add in the mint before scooping your breakfast into a bowl.

Nutritional facts: calories: 301, fats: 6 grams, carbohydrates: 57 grams, protein: 9 grams.

Coconut and Banana Mix

Time: 4 minutes

Servings: 4

Ingredients:

- 1 cup coconut milk
- 1 banana
- 1 cup dried coconut
- 2 tablespoons ground flax seed
- 3 tablespoons chopped raisins

- ⅛ teaspoon nutmeg
- ⅛ teaspoon cinnamon
- Salt to taste

Directions:

1. Set a large skillet on the stove and set it to low heat.
2. Chop up the banana.
3. Pour the coconut milk, nutmeg, and cinnamon into the skillet.
4. Pour in the ground flaxseed while stirring continuously.
5. Add the dried coconut and banana. Mix the ingredients until combined well.
6. Allow the mixture to simmer for 2 to 3 minutes while stirring occasionally.
7. Set four airtight containers on the counter.
8. Remove the pan from heat and sprinkle enough salt for your taste buds.
9. Divide the mixture into the containers and place them into the fridge overnight. They can remain in the fridge for up to 3 days.
10. Before you set this tasty mixture in the microwave to heat up, you need to let it thaw on the counter for a bit.

Nutritional facts: calories: 279, fats: 22 grams, carbohydrates: 25 grams, protein: 6.4 grams.

Honey Nut Granola

Time: 30 minutes

Servings: 6

Ingredients:

- ¼ cup honey
- 2 ½ cups rolled oats
- ¼ teaspoon sea salt
- 2 tablespoons ground flaxseed
- 2 teaspoons vanilla extract
- ⅓ cup chopped almonds
- ½ teaspoon ground cinnamon
- ¼ cup olive oil
- ½ cup dried apricots, chopped

Directions:

1. Set the temperature of your oven to 325 degrees Fahrenheit and line a baking pan with a piece of parchment paper. While you can grease the pan, it is easier to use parchment paper when you're cutting the granola.
2. Turn a burner on your stovetop to medium heat and add the salt, chopped almonds, cinnamon, and oats. Cook the mixture for 5 to 6 minutes while stirring occasionally.
3. Using a microwavable-safe dish, mix the flaxseed, apricots, oil, and honey. Set the mixture in your microwave and the timer for 1 minute. If the mixture does not bubble within the minute, continue

for another minute or until the mixture bubbles.
4. Mix the vanilla into the flaxseed mixture and then pour this mixture over the almond and oats mixture. Combine the ingredients thoroughly.
5. Remove the skillet from heat and pour onto the parchment paper. Spread the mixture as evenly as possible with a spatula or another sheet of parchment paper and your hand.
6. Set the pan into the oven and turn your timer to 15 minutes. However, you want to watch the granola closely as once it starts to brown, you'll need to remove it from heat.
7. Set the granola aside to cool thoroughly. If you used parchment paper, you can take the granola out of the pan by holding the paper and setting it on your counter. It will cool faster so you can eat it faster! Once this waiting is done, cut or break apart the granola into small pieces and enjoy!

Tip: Breaking apart the granola on the parchment paper makes for easy cleanup!

Nutritional facts: calories: 337, fats: 17 grams, carbohydrates: 42 grams, protein: 7 grams.

Cheese and Cauliflower Frittata With Peppers
Time: 30 minutes

Servings: 6

Ingredients:

- 10 eggs
- 1 seeded and chopped bell pepper
- ½ cup grated Parmigiano-Reggiano
- ½ cup milk, skim
- ½ teaspoon cayenne pepper
- 1 pound cauliflower, floret
- ½ teaspoon saffron
- 2 tablespoons chopped chives
- Salt and black pepper as desired

Directions:

1. Prepare your oven by setting the temperature to 370 degrees Fahrenheit. You should also grease a skillet suitable for the oven.
2. In a medium-sized bowl, add the milk and eggs. Whisk them until they are frothy.
3. Sprinkle the grated Parmigiano-Reggiano cheese into the frothy mixture and fold the ingredients together.
4. Pour in the salt, saffron, cayenne pepper, and black pepper and gently stir.
5. Add in the chopped bell pepper and gently stir until the ingredients are fully incorporated.
6. Pour the egg mixture into the skillet and cook on medium heat over your stovetop for 4 minutes.
7. Steam the cauliflower florets in a pan. To do this, add ½ inch of water and ½ teaspoon sea salt. Pour in the cauliflower and cover for 3 to 8 minutes. Drain any extra water.
8. Add the cauliflower into the mixture and gently stir.
9. Set the skillet into the preheated oven and turn

your timer to 13 minutes. Once the mixture is golden brown in the middle, remove the frittata from the oven.

10. Set your skillet aside for a couple of minutes so it can cool.
11. Slice and garnish with chives before you serve.

Nutritional facts: calories: 207, fats: 12 grams, carbohydrates: 8 grams, protein: 17 grams.

Omelet With Cheese and Broccoli

Time: 30 minutes

Servings: 4

Ingredients:

- 6 eggs
- 2 ½ cups of broccoli florets
- ¼ cup of milk
- 1 tablespoon olive oil
- ⅓ cup Romano cheese, grated
- ¼ teaspoon pepper
- ⅕ teaspoon salt
- ⅓ cup Greek olives, sliced
- Parsley and more Romano cheese for garnish

Directions:

1. Turn your oven to broil.
2. Set a steamer basket in a large pan and add 1 inch

of water.

3. Add the broccoli to the steamer basket and turn the range to medium. Once the water starts to boil, reduce the temperature to low. Steam the broccoli for 4 to 5 minutes. You will know the vegetable is done when it is soft and tender.
4. In a large bowl, whisk the eggs.
5. Pour in the milk, pepper, and salt.
6. Once the broccoli is done, toss into the large bowl and add the olives and grated cheese.
7. Grease an oven-proof 10-inch skillet and turn the heat on the burner to medium.
8. Add in the egg mixture, then cook for 4 to 5 minutes.
9. Set the skillet into the oven but make sure it's at least 4 inches from the heating source. Broil the eggs for 3 minutes. If the eggs are not completely set, continue cooking for another minute or two.
10. Remove the eggs from the oven and set on the stove so they can cool for a few minutes.
11. Garnish the omelet with cheese and parsley. Then, cut into wedges and enjoy!

Nutritional facts: calories: 229, fats: 17 grams, carbohydrates: 5 grams, protein: 15 grams.

Almond Pancakes

Time: 30 minutes

Servings: 6

Ingredients:

- ½ cup melted coconut oil, plus a little on the side for grease
- 2 cups unsweetened, room temperature almond milk
- 2 teaspoons raw honey
- 1 ½ cups whole wheat flour
- 2 eggs, room temperature
- ¼ teaspoon ground cinnamon
- ½ cup almond flour
- ¼ teaspoon sea salt
- ½ teaspoon baking soda
- 1 ½ teaspoons baking powder

Directions:

1. In a large bowl, whisk your eggs.
2. Add in the coconut oil, honey, and almond milk. Whisk thoroughly.
3. In a separate bowl, sift together your baking soda, baking powder, sea salt, almond flour, cinnamon, and whole wheat flour. Ensure the ingredients are well incorporated.
4. Combine the two mixtures by slowly adding your powdered ingredients into your wet ingredients. Stir as you combine as it will be easier to fully mix the ingredients.
5. Grease a large skillet with oil and set it on medium-high heat.
6. Using ½ cup measurements, pour the batter into

the skillet. Make sure the pancakes are not touching each other when they cook.

7. Let your pancakes cook for about 3 to 5 minutes on each side. Once bubbles start to break the surface and the edges become firm, flip the pancake over to cook the other side.
8. Once they are cooked thoroughly, place them on a plate and continue the process until all your batter is used up. You might need to grease your skillet again between batches.
9. To give your pancakes more of a Mediterranean flavor, add some fresh fruit on top.

Nutritional facts: calories: 286, fats: 17 grams, carbohydrates: 26 grams, protein: 7 grams.

Pear and Mango Smoothie

Time: 10 minutes

Servings: 1

Ingredients:

- ½ peeled, pitted, and chopped mango
- 2 cubes of ice
- 1 ripe, cored, and chopped pear
- ½ cup of plain Greek yogurt
- 1 cup chopped kale

Directions:

1. In a blender, combine the mango, ice cubes, pear, yogurt, and kale.

2. Blend until the mixture is smooth and thick.
3. Serve and enjoy!

Nutritional facts: calories: 293, fats: 8 grams, carbohydrates: 53 grams, protein: 8 grams.

Egg-Artichoke Breakfast Casserole
Time: 30 to 35 minutes

Servings: 8

Ingredients:
- 14 ounces artichoke hearts, if using canned remember to drain them
- 16 eggs
- 1 cup shredded cheddar cheese
- 10 ounces chopped spinach, if frozen make sure it is thawed and well-drained
- 1 clove of minced garlic
- ½ cup ricotta cheese
- ½ cup parmesan cheese
- ½ teaspoon crushed red pepper
- 1 teaspoon sea salt
- ½ teaspoon dried thyme
- ¼ cup onion, shaved
- ¼ cup milk

Directions:

1. Grease a 9 x 13-inch baking pan or place a piece of parchment paper inside of it.
2. Turn the temperature on your oven to 350 degrees Fahrenheit.
3. Crack the eggs into a bowl and whisk them well.
4. Pour in the milk and whisk the two ingredients together.
5. Squeeze any excess moisture from the spinach with a paper towel.
6. Toss the spinach and leafless artichoke hearts into the bowl. Stir until well combined.
7. Add the cheddar cheese, minced garlic, parmesan cheese, red pepper, sea salt, thyme, and onion into the bowl. Mix until all the ingredients are fully incorporated.
8. Pour the eggs into the baking pan.
9. Add the ricotta cheese in even dollops before placing the casserole in the oven.
10. Set your timer for 30 minutes, but watch the casserole carefully after about 20 minutes. Once the eggs stop jiggling and are cooked, remove the meal from the oven. Let the casserole cool down a bit and enjoy!

Nutritional facts: calories: 302, fats: 18 grams, carbohydrates: 11 grams, protein: 22 grams.

Breakfast Burrito Mediterranean Style

Time: 20 minutes

Servings: 6 burritos

Ingredients:

- 9 eggs
- 3 tablespoons chopped sun-dried tomatoes
- 6 tortillas that are 10 inches
- 2 cups baby spinach
- ½ cup feta cheese
- ¾ cups of canned refried beans
- 3 tablespoons sliced black olives
- Salsa, sour cream, or any other toppings you desire

Directions:

1. Wash and dry your spinach.
2. Grease a medium frying pan with oil or nonstick cooking spray.
3. Add the eggs into the pan and cook for about 5 minutes. Make sure you stir the eggs well, so they become scrambled.
4. Combine the black olives, spinach, and sun-dried tomatoes with the eggs. Stir until the ingredients are fully incorporated.
5. Add the feta cheese and then set the lid on the pan so the cheese will melt quickly.
6. Spoon a bit of egg mixture into the tortilla.
7. Wrap the tortillas tightly.
8. Wash your pan or get a new skillet. Remember to grease the pan.
9. Set each tortilla into the pan and cook each side for

a couple of minutes. Once they are lightly brown, remove them from the pan and allow the burritos to cool on a serving plate. Top with your favorite condiments and enjoy!
10. To store the burritos, wrap them in aluminum foil and place them in the fridge. They can be stored for up to two days.

Nutritional facts: calories: 252, fats: 11 grams, carbohydrates: 21 grams, protein: 14 grams.

Ham and Egg Muffins

Time: 25 minutes

Servings: 6 muffins

Ingredients:

- ¼ cup crumbled feta cheese
- ⅛ teaspoon salt
- 1 ½ tablespoons of pesto sauce
- 9 slices of deli ham
- ⅓ cup chopped spinach
- 5 eggs
- ⅛ teaspoon of pepper
- ½ cup roasted red pepper plus a little for garnish
- Basil for garnish

Directions:

1. Turn the temperature on your oven to 400 degrees Fahrenheit.

2. Grease the cups of the muffin tin.
3. Line each muffin tin cup with a slice of ham. The trick is to ensure there are no holes within the ham so none of the egg mixture seeps out.
4. Add some roasted peppers into the muffin cup.
5. Add 1 tablespoon of chopped spinach on top of the roasted pepper.
6. Sprinkle ½ tablespoon of feta cheese on top of the spinach.
7. Combine the eggs in a bowl with the salt and pepper. Whisk well.
8. Divide the egg mixture evenly between the 6 muffin tins.
9. Set in your oven and turn the timer for 15 minutes. If the eggs are not set and puffy after 15 minutes, keep them in the oven for another minute or two.
10. Carefully remove the muffins from the muffin tin cups and let them cool completely.
11. Garnish and enjoy your breakfast muffins, or you can store them in the fridge for up to three days. To warm them up, microwave them for 30 seconds.

Nutritional facts: calories: 109, fats: 6 grams, carbohydrates: 2 grams, protein: 9 grams.

Thick Pomegranate Cherry Smoothie

Time: 5 minutes

Servings: 4

Ingredients:

- 16 ounces frozen dark cherries
- ¾ cup pomegranate juice
- 1 teaspoon vanilla extract
- 6 ice cubes
- ½ cup pomegranate seeds
- 1 ½ cups Greek yogurt, plain
- ⅓ cup milk
- ¾ teaspoon ground cinnamon
- ½ cup pistachios, chopped

Directions:

1. Add the ice cubes, cherries, pomegranate juice, yogurt, vanilla, milk, and cinnamon into a blender. Mix until the ingredients are smooth. It is thicker than your average smoothie.
2. Instead of a cup, divide the smoothie into four bowls.
3. Sprinkle chopped pistachios and pomegranate seeds on top of the smoothie.
4. Serve and enjoy!

Nutritional facts: calories: 212, fats: 7 grams, carbohydrates: 35 grams, protein: 4 grams.

Lunch

Delicious Broccoli Tortellini Salad
Time: 20 to 25 minutes

Servings: 12

Ingredients:

- 1 cup sunflower seeds, or any of your favorite seeds
- 3 heads of broccoli, fresh is best!
- ½ cup sugar
- 20 ounces cheese-filled tortellini
- 1 onion
- 2 teaspoons cider vinegar
- ½ cup mayonnaise
- 1 cup raisins-optional

Directions:

1. Cut your broccoli into florets and chop the onion.
2. Follow the directions to make the cheese-filled tortellini. Once they are cooked, drain and rinse them with cold water.
3. In a bowl, combine your mayonnaise, sugar, and vinegar. Whisk well to give the ingredients a dressing consistency.
4. In a separate large bowl, toss in your seeds, onion, tortellini, raisins, and broccoli.
5. Pour the salad dressing into the large bowl and toss the ingredients together. You will want to ensure everything is thoroughly mixed as you'll want a taste of the salad dressing with every bite!

Nutritional facts: calories: 272, fats: 8.1 grams, carbohydrates: 38.6 grams, protein: 5 grams.

Grilled Lemon Fish

Time: 15 minutes

Servings: 4

Ingredients:

- ¼ teaspoon sea salt
- 3 to 4 lemons
- ¼ teaspoon ground black pepper
- 4 ounces any fish fillets, such as salmon or cod
- 1 tablespoon olive oil

Directions:

1. Ensure that the fish fillets are dry. If you know or feel they are a bit damp, take a paper towel and pat them dry.
2. Leave the fish fillets on the counter for 10 minutes so they can stand at room temperature.
3. Turn on your grill to medium-high heat or set the temperature to 400 degrees Fahrenheit.
4. Using nonstick cooking spray, coat the grill so the fish won't stick.
5. Take one lemon and cut it in half. Set one of the halves aside and cut the remaining half into ¼-inch thick slices.
6. Now, take the other half of the lemon and squeeze at least 1 tablespoon of juice out into a small bowl.
7. Add oil into the small bowl and whisk the

ingredients together.

8. Brush the fish with the lemon and oil mixture. Make sure you get both sides of the fish.
9. Arrange the lemon slices on the grill in the shape of the fish, it might take about 3 to 4 slices for one fish.
10. Place the fish on top of the lemon slices and grill the ingredients together. If you don't have a lid for your grill, cover it with a different lid that will fit or use aluminum foil.
11. When the fish is about half-way done, turn it over so the other side is laying on top of the lemon slices.
12. You will know the fish is done when it starts to look flaky and separates easily, which you can check by gently pressing a fork onto the fish.

Nutritional facts: calories: 147, fats: 5 grams, carbohydrates: 4 grams, protein: 22 grams.

Chicken Drummies With Peach Glaze

Time: 25 minutes

Servings: 4

Ingredients:

- 2 pounds of chicken drummies, remove the skin
- 15 ounce can of sliced peaches, drain the juice
- ¼ cup cider vinegar
- ½ teaspoon paprika
- ¼ teaspoon black pepper

- ¼ cup honey
- 3 garlic cloves
- ¼ teaspoon sea salt

Directions:

1. Before you turn your oven on, make sure that one rack is 4 inches below the broiler element.
2. Set your oven's temperature to 500 degrees Fahrenheit.
3. Line a large baking sheet with a piece of aluminum foil.
4. Set a wire cooling rack on top of the foil.
5. Spray the rack with cooking spray.
6. Add the honey, peaches, garlic, vinegar, salt, paprika, and pepper into a blender. Mix until smooth.
7. Set a medium saucepan on top of your stove and set the range temperature to medium heat.
8. Pour the mixture into the saucepan and bring it to a boil while stirring constantly.
9. Once the sauce is done, divide it into two small bowls and set one off to the side.
10. With the second bowl, brush half of the mixture onto the chicken drummies.
11. Roast the drummies for 10 minutes.
12. Take the drummies out of the oven and switch to broiler mode.
13. Brush the drummies with the other half of the sauce from the second bowl.

14. Again, place the drummies back into the oven and set a timer for 5 minutes.
15. When the timer goes off, flip the drummies over and broil for another 3 to 4 minutes.
16. Serve the drummies with the reserved sauce and enjoy!

Nutritional facts: calories: 291, fats: 5 grams, carbohydrates: 33 grams, protein: 30 grams.

Mediterranean Potato Salad

Time: 30 minutes

Servings: 6

Ingredients:

- 3 tablespoons extra virgin olive oil
- ½ cup of sliced olives
- 1 tablespoon olive juice
- 3 tablespoons lemon juice, freshly squeezed is best
- 2 tablespoons of mint, fresh and torn
- ¼ teaspoon sea salt
- 2 stalks of sliced celery
- 2 pounds baby potatoes
- 2 tablespoons of chopped oregano, fresh is best

Directions:

1. Cut the potatoes into 1-inch cubes.
2. Toss the potatoes into a medium saucepan and

cover them with water.
3. Place the saucepan on the stove over high heat.
4. Once the potatoes start to boil, bring the heat down to medium-low.
5. Let the potatoes simmer for 13 to 15 minutes. When you poke the potatoes with a fork and they feel tender, they are done.
6. As the potatoes are simmering, grab a small bowl and mix the oil, olive juice, lemon juice, and salt. Whisk the ingredients together well.
7. Once the potatoes are done, drain them and pour the potatoes into a bowl.
8. Take the juice mixture and pour 3 tablespoons over the potatoes right away.
9. Combine the potatoes with the celery and olives.
10. Prior to serving, sprinkle the potatoes with the mint, oregano, and rest of the dressing.

Nutritional facts: calories: 175, fats: 7 grams, carbohydrates: 27 grams, protein: 3 grams.

Bean Lettuce Wraps

Time: 20 minutes

Servings: 4

Ingredients:

- 8 Romaine lettuce leaves
- ½ cup Garlic hummus or any prepared hummus
- ¾ cup chopped tomatoes
- 15 ounce can great northern beans, drained and

rinsed
- ½ cup diced onion
- 1 tablespoon extra virgin olive oil
- ¼ cup chopped parsley
- ¼ teaspoon black pepper

Directions:

1. Set a skillet on top of the stove range over medium heat.
2. In the skillet, warm the oil for a couple of minutes.
3. Add the onion into the oil. Stir frequently as the onion cooks for a few minutes.
4. Combine the pepper and tomatoes and cook for another couple of minutes. Remember to stir occasionally.
5. Add the beans and continue to stir and cook for 2 to 3 minutes.
6. Turn the burner off, remove the skillet from heat, and add the parsley.
7. Set the lettuce leaves on a flat surface and spread 1 tablespoon of hummus on each leaf.
8. Divide the bean mixture onto the 8 leaves.
9. Spread the bean mixture down the center of the leaves.
10. Fold the leaves by starting lengthwise on one side.
11. Fold over the other side so the leaf is completely wrapped.
12. Serve and enjoy!

Nutritional facts: calories: 211, fats: 8 grams, carbohydrates: 28 grams, protein: 10 grams.

Tuna Bowl With Kale

Time: 15 to 20 minutes

Servings: 6

Ingredients:

- 3 tablespoons extra virgin olive oil
- 1 ½ teaspoons minced garlic
- ¼ cup of capers
- 2 teaspoons sugar
- 15 ounce can of drained and rinsed great northern beans
- 1 pound chopped kale with the center ribs removed
- ½ teaspoon ground black pepper
- 1 cup chopped onion
- 2 ½ ounces of drained sliced olives
- ¼ teaspoon sea salt
- ¼ teaspoon crushed red pepper
- 6 ounces of tuna in olive oil, do not drain

Directions:

1. Place a large pot, like a stockpot, on your stove and turn the burner to high heat.
2. Fill the pot about 3-quarters of the way full with water and let it come to a boil.
3. Add the kale and cook for 2 minutes.
4. Drain the kale and set it aside.
5. Turn the heat down to medium and place the empty pot back on the burner.

6. Add the oil and onion. Saute for 3 to 4 minutes.
7. Combine the garlic into the oil mixture and saute for another minute.
8. Add the capers, olives, and red pepper.
9. Cook the ingredients for another minute while stirring.
10. Pour in the sugar and stir while you toss in the kale. Mix all the ingredients thoroughly and ensure the kale is thoroughly coated.
11. Cover the pot and set the timer for 8 minutes.
12. Turn off the heat and add in the tuna, pepper, beans, salt, and any other herbs that will make this one of the best Mediterranean dishes you've ever made.

Nutritional facts: calories: 265, fats: 12 grams, carbohydrates: 26 grams, protein: 16 grams.

Italian Tuna Sandwiches

Time: 10 minutes

Servings: 4

Ingredients:

- 3 tablespoons lemon juice, freshly squeezed
- ½ teaspoon of minced garlic
- 5 ounces tuna, drained
- ½ cup of sliced olives
- 8 slices whole-grain bread
- 2 tablespoons extra virgin olive oil

- ½ teaspoon black pepper
- 1 celery stalk, chopped

Directions:

1. Add the oil, pepper, lemon juice, and garlic to a bowl. Whisk the ingredients well.
2. Combine the olives, chopped celery, and tuna.
3. Use a fork to break apart the tuna into chunks.
4. Stir all of the ingredients until they are well combined.
5. Set four slices of bread on serving plates or a platter.
6. Divide the tuna salad equally among the four slices of bread.
7. Top the tuna salad with the remaining bread to make a sandwich.
8. You'll get the best taste when you let the tuna sandwich sit for about 5 or more minutes before you serve. The salad will start to soak into the bread, and it makes for one tasty meal!

Nutritional facts: calories: 347, fats: 17 grams, carbohydrates: 27 grams, protein: 25 grams.

Flatbread With Roasted Vegetables

Time: 45 minutes

Servings: 12 slices

Ingredients:

- 5 ounces goat cheese

- 1 thinly sliced onion
- 2 thinly sliced tomatoes
- Olive oil
- ¼ teaspoon pepper
- ⅛ teaspoon salt
- 16 ounces homemade or frozen pizza dough
- ¾ tablespoon chopped dill, fresh is better
- 1 thinly sliced zucchini
- 1 red pepper, cup into rings

Directions:

1. Set your oven to 400 degrees Fahrenheit.
2. Set the dough on a large piece of parchment paper. Use a rolling pin to roll the dough into a large rectangle.
3. Spread half of the goat cheese on ½ of the pizza dough.
4. Sprinkle half of the dill on the other half of the dough.
5. Fold the dough so the half with the dill is on top of the cheese.
6. Spread the remaining goat cheese on the pizza dough and then sprinkle the rest of the dill over the cheese.
7. Layer the vegetables on top in any arrangement you like.
8. Drizzle olive oil on top of the vegetables.
9. Sprinkle salt and pepper over the olive oil.
10. Set the piece of parchment paper on a pizza pan or

baking pan and place it in the oven.
11. Set the timer for 22 minutes. If the edges are not a medium brown, leave the flatbread in the oven for another couple of minutes.
12. Remove the pizza from the oven when it is done and cut the flatbread in half lengthwise.
13. Slice the flatbread into 2-inch long pieces and enjoy!

Nutritional facts: calories: 170, fats: 5 grams, carbohydrates: 20 grams, protein: 8 grams.

Steamed Mussels Topped With Wine Sauce

Time: 15 minutes

Servings: 4

Ingredients:

- 2 pounds mussels
- 1 tablespoon extra virgin olive oil
- 1 cup sliced onion
- 1 cup dry white wine
- ¼ teaspoon ground black pepper
- ¼ teaspoon sea salt
- 3 sliced cloves of garlic
- 2 lemon slices
- Optional: lemon wedges for serving

Directions:

1. Set a large colander in the sink and turn your water

to cold.
2. Run water over the mussels, but do not let them sit in the water. If you notice any shells that are not tightly sealed or are cracked, you need to discard them. All shells need to be closed tightly.
3. Turn off the water and leave the mussels in the colander.
4. Set a large skillet on your stovetop and turn your range heat to medium-high.
5. Pour the olive oil into the skillet and allow it to heat up before you add the onion.
6. Saute the onion for 2 to 3 minutes.
7. Combine the garlic and cook the mixture for another minute while stirring continuously.
8. Pour in the wine, pepper, lemon slices, and salt. Stir the ingredients as you bring them to a boil.
9. Add the mussels and place the lid on the skillet.
10. Cook the mixture for 3 to 4 minutes or until the shells begin to open on the mussels. It will help to gently pick up the skillet and shake it a couple of times when the mussels are cooking.
11. If you notice any shells that did not open, use a spoon and discard them.
12. Scoop the mussels into a serving bowl and pour the mixture over the top.
13. If you have lemon wedges, place them on the top of the steamed mussels before serving. Enjoy!

Nutritional facts: calories: 222, fats: 7 grams, carbohydrates: 11 grams, protein: 18 grams.

Carrot Soup With Parmesan Croutons

Time: 25 to 30 minutes

Servings: 4

Ingredients:

- 2 cups vegetable broth, no salt added, and low sodium is best
- 1 teaspoon dried thyme
- ¼ teaspoon sea salt
- 1 ounce grated parmesan cheese
- 2 pounds of carrots, unpeeled
- 2 tablespoons extra virgin olive oil
- ½ chopped onion
- 2 ½ cups water
- ¼ teaspoon crushed red pepper
- 4 slices of whole-grain bread

Directions:

1. Cut your carrots into ½-inch slices
2. Take one rack from your oven and place it four inches from the broiler heating element.
3. One either rack, place two large-rimmed baking sheets and turn your oven to 450 degrees Fahrenheit.
4. Add 1 tablespoon of oil and carrots into a large bowl. Stir the carrots around so they become coated with the oil.
5. Using oven mitts, remove the baking pans and distribute the carrots onto them.
6. Place the pans back into the oven and turn your

timer on for 20 minutes or until the carrots become tender.
7. Take the carrots out of the oven.
8. Turn your oven to broiler mode.
9. Set a large stockpot on your stove and turn the range to medium-high.
10. Pour in the remaining olive oil and the onion. Let it cook for 5 minutes while stirring occasionally.
11. Pour in the broth, thyme, water, crushed red pepper, and sea salt. Stir well.
12. Let the mixture cook until the ingredients come to a boil.
13. Once the carrots are done in the oven, add them to the pot.
14. Remove the pot from the heat and carefully pour the soup into a blender. You will want to pour it in batches and remember to hold the lid of the blender with a rag and release the steam after 30 seconds, so it doesn't explode.
15. Once all the soup is mixed, add it all back into the pot and turn the range heat to medium. Cook until the soup is warm again.
16. Spread a piece of parchment paper on top of a baking sheet, set the four pieces of bread on the paper.
17. Sprinkle cheese across the slices and set them on the top rack in your oven.
18. Turn your oven to broil and let the slices of bread roast for a couple of minutes. Once the cheese is melted, remove the bread from the oven so they don't burn.

19. Chop the bread into croutons.
20. Divide the soup into serving bowls, add the croutons, and enjoy!

Nutritional facts: calories: 272, fats: 10 grams, carbohydrates: 38 grams, protein: 10 grams.

Dinner

Spinach and Beans Mediterranean Style Salad

Time: 30 minutes

Servings: 4

Ingredients:

- 15 ounces drained and rinsed cannellini beans
- 14 ounces drained, rinsed, and quartered artichoke hearts
- 6 ounces or 8 cups baby spinach
- 14 ½ ounces undrained diced tomatoes, no salt is best
- 1 tablespoon olive oil and any additional if you prefer
- ¼ teaspoon salt
- 2 minced garlic cloves
- 1 chopped onion, small in size
- ¼ teaspoon pepper
- ⅛ teaspoon crushed red pepper flakes
- 2 tablespoons Worcestershire sauce

Directions:

1. Place a saucepan on your stovetop and turn the temperature to medium-high.
2. Let the pan warm up for a minute before you pour in the tablespoon of oil. Continue to let the oil heat up for another minute or two.
3. Toss in your chopped onion and stir so all the pieces are bathed in oil. Saute the onions for 3 minutes.
4. Add the garlic to the saucepan. Stir and saute the ingredients for another minute.
5. Combine the salt, red pepper flakes, pepper, and Worcestershire sauce. Mix well and then add the tomatoes to the pan. Stir the mixture constantly for about 5 minutes.
6. Add the artichoke hearts, spinach, and beans. Saute and stir occasionally to get the taste throughout the dish. Once the spinach starts to wilt, take the salad off of the heat.
7. Serve and enjoy immediately to get the best taste.

Nutritional facts: calories: 187, fats: 4 grams, carbohydrates: 30 grams, protein: 8 grams.

Lasagna

Time: 1 hour 15 minutes

Servings: 8

Ingredients:

- Lasagna noodles, oven-ready are the best, easiest, and quickest
- ⅓ cup flour
- 2 tablespoons chives, divided and chopped
- ½ cup white wine
- 2 tablespoons olive oil
- 1 ½ tablespoons thyme
- 1 teaspoon salt
- 1 ¼ cups shallots, chopped
- 1 cup boiled water
- ½ cup Parmigiano-Reggiano cheese
- 3 cups milk, reduced-fat and divided
- 1 tablespoon butter
- ⅓ cup cream cheese, less fat is the best choice
- 6 cloves of garlic, divided and minced
- ½ teaspoon ground black pepper, divided
- 4 ounces dried shiitake mushrooms, sliced
- 1 ounce dried porcini mushrooms, sliced
- 8 ounces cremini mushrooms, sliced

Directions:

1. Keeping your mushrooms separated, drain them all and return them to separate containers.
2. Bring 1 cup of water to a boil and cook your porcini mushrooms for a half hour.
3. Preheat your oven to 350 degrees Fahrenheit.
4. Set a large pan on your stove and turn the burner to medium-high heat.
5. Add your butter and let it melt.

6. Combine the olive oil and shallots. Stir the mixture and let it cook for 3 minutes.
7. Pour half of the pepper, half of the salt, and mushrooms into the pan. Allow the mixture to cook for 6 to 7 minutes.
8. While stirring, add half of the garlic and thyme. Continue to stir for 1 minute.
9. Pour the wine and turn your burner temperature to high. Let the mixture boil and watch the liquid evaporate for a couple of minutes to reduce it slightly.
10. Turn off the burner and remove the pan from heat.
11. Add the cream cheese and chives. Stir thoroughly.
12. Set a medium-sized skillet on medium-high heat and add 1 tablespoon of oil. Let the oil come to a simmer.
13. Add the last of the garlic to the pan and saute for 30 seconds.
14. Pour in 2 ⅓ cup milk and the liquid from the porcini mushrooms. Stir the mixture and allow it to boil.
15. In a bowl, combine ¼ cup of milk and the flour. Add this mixture to the heated pan. Stir until the mixture starts to thicken.
16. Grease a pan and add ½ cup of sauce along with a row of noodles.
17. Spread half of the mushroom mixture on top of the noodles.
18. Repeat the process, but make sure you top the lasagna with mushrooms and cheese.
19. Turn your timer to 45 minutes and set the pan into the oven.

20. Remember to garnish the lasagna with chives before enjoying!

Nutritional facts: calories: 268, fats: 12.6 grams, carbohydrates: 29 grams, protein: 10 grams.

Salmon Skillet Dinner

Time: 15 to 20 minutes

Servings: 4

Ingredients:

- 1 teaspoon minced garlic
- 1 ½ cup quartered cherry tomatoes
- 1 tablespoon water
- ¼ teaspoon sea salt
- 1 tablespoon lemon juice, freshly squeezed is best
- 1 tablespoon extra virgin olive oil
- 12 ounces drained and chopped roasted red peppers
- 1 teaspoon paprika
- ¼ teaspoon black pepper
- 1 pound salmon fillets

Directions:

1. Remove the skin from your salmon fillets and cut them into 8 pieces.
2. Turn your stove burner on medium heat and set a skillet on top.
3. Pour the olive oil into the skillet and let it heat up for a couple of minutes.

4. Add the minced garlic and paprika. Saute the ingredients for 1 minute.
5. Combine the roasted peppers, black pepper, tomatoes, water, and salt.
6. Set the heat to medium-high and bring the ingredients to a simmer. This should take 3 to 4 minutes. Remember to stir the ingredients occasionally so the tomatoes don't burn.
7. Add the salmon and take some of the sauce from the skillet to spoon on top of the fish so it is all covered in the mixture.
8. Cover the skillet and set a timer for 10 minutes. When the fish reaches 145 degrees Fahrenheit, it is cooked thoroughly.
9. Turn off the heat and drizzle lemon juice over the fish.
10. Break up the salmon into chunks and gently mix the pieces of fish with the sauce.
11. Serve and enjoy!

Nutritional facts: calories: 289, fats: 13 grams, carbohydrates: 10 grams, protein: 31 grams.

Barley and Mushroom Soup

Time: 3o minutes

Servings: 6

Ingredients:

- 2 tablespoons of olive oil
- 1 cup chopped carrots

- 6 cups vegetable broth, no salt added, and low sodium is best
- ¼ cup red wine
- 5 tablespoons parmesan cheese, grated
- ½ teaspoon thyme
- 1 cup chopped onion
- 5 cups chopped mushrooms
- 1 cup pearled barley, uncooked
- 2 tablespoons tomato paste

Directions:

1. Place a stockpot on your stove and turn the temperature of the range to medium heat.
2. Pour in the oil and let it warm up and start to simmer.
3. Combine the carrots and onion. Let them cook for 5 to 8 minutes while frequently stirring the ingredients together.
4. Add the mushroom and turn the heat up to medium-high. Stir and cook for a few minutes.
5. Pour in the broth and stir the ingredients for a few seconds.
6. Add in the wine, barley, thyme, and tomato paste. Stir everything together and then set the cover on the pot.
7. When the soup starts to boil, stir and reduce the heat to medium-low.
8. Cover the soup again and set your timer for 15 minutes, but don't leave it alone. You will want to

stir a few times, so all ingredients become well incorporated.
9. Once the dish becomes fragrant and the barley is completely cooked, turn off the heat and serve in bowls. Sprinkle the cheese on top for added taste and enjoy!

Nutritional facts: calories: 236, fats: 7 grams, carbohydrates: 35 grams, protein: 8 grams.

Seafood Paella

Time: 1 hour

Servings: 4 to 5

Ingredients:

- 4 lobster tails that should be around 6 to 12 ounces each
- 3 tablespoons extra virgin olive oil
- 2 cups short-grain rice
- 1 tablespoon paprika
- ½ teaspoon red pepper flakes
- 2 finely chopped tomatoes
- 1 chopped onion
- 1 pound peeled and deveined shrimp
- 4 chopped garlic cloves
- 1 teaspoon cayenne pepper
- ¼ cup chopped parsley
- 5 ounces of trimmed french green beans
- 3 cups of water

Directions:

1. Soak the rice in water for 15 to 20 minutes and then drain.
2. Turn one of the ranges on your stove to high heat and then boil a pot with water.
3. Carefully add the lobster tails to the water and boil them for 2 to 3 minutes. Once they become pink, use tongs to remove them from the heat and transfer to plates.
4. Turn off the heat, but keep the water in the pot.
5. Once the lobster is cool, remove the shell and cut the seafood into large chunks.
6. Place a skillet on a burner and turn to medium-high heat.
7. Pour 3 tablespoons of olive oil into the skillet.
8. Once the oil is warm, saute the onions for 2 minutes.
9. Combine the rice and cook the ingredients for 3 to 4 minutes while stirring often.
10. Pour the lobster water into the skillet and add the garlic, red pepper flakes, cayenne pepper, and paprika. Mix well.
11. Add in the green beans and tomatoes. Stir all the ingredients until they come to a boil.
12. Reduce the heat to low, cover, and let the mixture cook for 20 minutes.
13. Once most of the liquid is absorbed, lay the shrimp on top of the mixture. If the rice looks too dry, add a little more water.
14. Cover and set the timer for another 15 minutes, but

watch the shrimp. Once it turns pink, you will add in the lobster chunks.
15. Let the lobster warm up in the skillet.
16. Turn off the heat and remove the skillet from the burner. Plate and enjoy!

Nutritional facts: calories: 536, fats: 25 grams, carbohydrates: 56 grams, protein: 51 grams.

Italian Baked Beans

Time: 15 to 20 minutes.

Servings: 6

Ingredients:

- ½ cup chopped onion
- ¼ cup red wine vinegar
- ¼ tablespoon ground cinnamon
- 15 ounces or 2 cans of great northern beans, do not drain
- 2 teaspoons extra virgin olive oil
- 12 ounces tomato paste, low sodium
- ½ cup water

Directions:

1. Turn a burner to medium heat and add oil to a saucepan.
2. Add the onion and cook for 4 to 5 minutes. Stir well.
3. Combine the vinegar, tomato paste, cinnamon, and water. Mix until all the ingredients are well

combined.
4. Switch the heat to a low setting.
5. Using a colander, drain one can of beans and pour into the pan.
6. Open the second can of beans and pour all of it, including the liquid, into the saucepan and stir.
7. Continue to cook the beans for 10 minutes while stirring frequently.
8. Serve and enjoy!

Nutritional facts: calories: 236, fats: 3 grams, carbohydrates: 42 grams, protein: 10 grams.

Chickpeas and Brussel Sprouts Salad

Time: 10 minutes

Servings: 4

Ingredients:

- 1 cup roasted chickpeas. To give the dish a saltier taste, you can add sea salt.
- 4 cups kale, chopped
- 9 ounces Brussels sprouts, shredded
- 1 avocado, peeled, pitted, and cut

Directions:

1. Divide the kale and Brussels sprouts into four bowls.
2. Add the chickpeas and the avocado.
3. You can add a little sea salt and/or pepper to taste. Another tip for more taste is to drizzle a little

Vinaigrette dressing or your favorite homemade Mediterranean dressing.

Nutritional facts: calories: 337, fats: 20 grams, carbohydrates: 30 grams, protein: 12 grams.

Vegetarian Lasagna Roll-Ups

Time: 1 hour 10 minutes

Servings: 14

Ingredients:

- 1 pound lasagna noodles
- 3 thinly sliced zucchini, if your vegetables are smaller make it 4
- ½ cup water
- 3 tablespoons olive oil
- Parmesan cheese and salt to taste
- 24-ounce jar of pasta sauce, you can use any type but the best for the recipes is basil or tomato
- Enough crushed red pepper flakes for your taste buds, this is also optional

For the cheese filling:

- 6 ounces goat cheese
- 20 ounces of ricotta cheese
- 2 ounces mozzarella cheese
- 1 cup of parsley leaves, chopped
- Dash of salt and pepper
- 3 tablespoons of chopped garlic
- Olive oil

Directions:

1. Set the temperature of your oven to 450 degrees Fahrenheit.
2. Grease a baking sheet or lay a piece of parchment paper on top.
3. Slice the zucchini and place them on the baking sheet.
4. Brush each side of the vegetable with oil and then sprinkle with salt.
5. Place the baking sheet into the oven and set a timer for 10 minutes.
6. While the zucchini is baking, start boiling the lasagna noodles. Drain the noodles when they are done cooking and then let them dry on a piece of parchment paper.
7. Remove the zucchini from the oven and set aside to allow them to cool down a bit.
8. Change the heat of your oven to 350 degrees Fahrenheit.
9. To make the cheese filling, combine all of the ingredients and drizzle with a little olive oil. Mix well.
10. Pour a spoonful or two on each of the lasagna noodles.
11. Set a slice of baked zucchini on top of the cheese mixture.
12. Roll up the noodles.

13. In a 9 x 13-inch baking pan, pour the water and ¾ cup of the pasta sauce on the bottom. Stir the ingredients gently so they become mixed.
14. Place the lasagna roll-ups in the upright position on top of the sauce.
15. Pour the remaining sauce on the noodles.
16. If you want a little extra cheese, sprinkle some on top of the lasagna roll-ups.
17. Set your timer for 40 minutes, but remember to check the liquid half-way through cooking to make sure it does not become too dry. If it does, add a little more water. You can try adding some water to the pasta sauce jar and shaking it up a bit as this will give the water a little sauce flavor.
18. When the lasagna is cooked, remove it and garnish with basil leaves. Allow it to cool for a couple of minutes and admire your Mediterranean cooking skills before serving.

Nutritional facts: calories: 282, fats: 11 grams, carbohydrates: 29 grams, protein: 14.3 grams.

Mediterranean Pizza

Time: 20 minutes

Servings: 4 to 8

Ingredients:

- 1/2 cup artichoke hearts
- Whole-wheat premade pizza crust
- 1 cup pesto sauce

- 1 cup spinach leaves
- 3 to 4 ounces of feta cheese
- 1 cup sun-dried tomatoes
- 3 ounces of mozzarella cheese
- ½ cup of olives
- Olive oil
- ½ cup bell peppers
- Chopped chicken, pepperoni, or salami

Directions:

1. Turn the temperature of your oven to 350 degrees Fahrenheit.
2. Use olive oil to brush the top of the whole wheat pizza crust.
3. Brush the pesto sauce on the pizza crust.
4. Top with all of the ingredients. You can start with the cheese or mix the ingredients in any way you wish. You can even get a little creative and have fun.
5. Set your pizza on a pizza pan or directly on your oven rack.
6. Set your timer to 10 minutes, but watch the pizza carefully so you do not burn the cheese.
7. Remove the pizza and let it cool down for a couple of minutes, then enjoy!

Nutritional facts: calories: 300, fats: 11 grams, carbohydrates: 29 grams, protein: 14 grams.

Garlic and Cajun Shrimp Bowl With Noodles

Time: 15 minutes

Servings: 2

Ingredients:

- 1 sliced onion
- 1 tablespoon almond butter, but you can use regular butter as well
- 1 teaspoon onion powder
- ½ teaspoon salt
- 1 sliced red pepper
- 3 cloves of minced garlic
- 1 teaspoon paprika
- 20 jumbo shrimp, deveined and shells removed
- 3 tablespoons of ghee
- 2 zucchini, 3 if they are smaller in size, cut into noodles
- Red pepper flakes and cayenne pepper, as desired

Directions:

1. In a small bowl, mix the pepper flakes, paprika, onion powder, salt, and cayenne pepper.
2. Toss the shrimp into the cajun mixture and coat the seafood thoroughly.
3. Add the ghee to a medium or large skillet and place on medium-low heat.
4. Once the ghee is melted, add the garlic and saute for 4 minutes.
5. Carefully add the shrimp into the skillet and cook until they are opaque. Set the pan aside.
6. In a new pan, add the butter and allow it to melt.

7. Combine the zucchini noodles and cook on medium-low heat for 3 to 4 minutes.
8. Turn off the heat and place the zucchini noodles on serving dishes. Add the shrimp to the top and enjoy.

Nutritional facts: calories: 712, fats: 30 grams, carbohydrates: 20.1 grams, protein: 98 grams.

Grilled Calamari With Berries

Time: 5 minutes

Servings: 4

Ingredients:

- ¼ cup olive oil
- ¼ cup extra virgin olive oil
- 1 thinly sliced apple
- ¾ cup blueberries
- ¼ cup sliced almonds
- 1 ½ pounds calamari tube
- ¼ cup dried cranberries
- 6 cups spinach
- 2 tablespoons apple cider vinegar
- 1 tablespoon lemon juice
- Sea salt and pepper to your liking

Directions:

1. Start by making the vinaigrette. Combine apple cider vinegar, lemon juice, extra virgin olive oil, sea salt, and pepper. Whisk well and set aside.
2. Set your grill to medium heat.
3. In a separate bowl, add the calamari tube and mix with salt, pepper, and olive oil.
4. Set the calamari on the grill and cook both sides for 2 to 3 minutes.
5. In another bowl, mix the salad by adding the spinach, cranberries, almonds, blueberries, and apples. Toss to mix.
6. Set the cooked calamari onto a cutting board and let it cool for a few minutes. Cut them into ¼-inch thick rings and then toss them into the salad bowl.
7. Sprinkle the vinaigrette sauce onto the salad. Toss to mix the ingredients and enjoy!

Nutritional facts: calories: 567, fats: 24.4 grams, carbohydrates: 30 grams, protein: 55 grams.

Dessert

Chocolate Fruit Kebabs

Time: 30 minutes

Servings: 6

Ingredients:

- 24 blueberries
- 12 strawberries with the green leafy top part removed
- 12 green or red grapes, seedless
- 12 pitted cherries
- 8 ounces chocolate

Directions:

1. Line a baking sheet with a piece of parchment paper and place 6, 12-inch long wooden skewers on top of the paper.
2. Start by threading a piece of fruit onto the skewers. You can create and follow any pattern that you like with the ingredients. An example pattern is 1 strawberry, 1 cherry, 2 blueberries, 2 grapes. Repeat the pattern until all of the fruit is on the skewers.
3. In a saucepan on medium heat, melt the chocolate. Stir continuously until the chocolate has melted completely.
4. Carefully scoop the chocolate into a plastic sandwich bag and twist the bag closed starting right above the chocolate.
5. Snip the corner of the bag with scissors.
6. Drizzle the chocolate onto the kebabs by squeezing it out of the bag.
7. Put the baking pan into the freezer for 20 minutes.
8. Serve and enjoy!

Nutritional facts: calories: 254, fats: 15 grams, carbohydrates: 28 grams, protein: 4 grams.

A Lemony Treat

Time: 30 minutes, including chill time

Servings: 4

Ingredients:

- 1 lemon, medium in size
- 1 ½ teaspoons cornstarch
- 1 cup Greek yogurt, plain is best
- Fresh fruit
- ¼ cup cold water
- ⅔ cup heavy whipped cream
- 3 tablespoons honey
- Optional: mint leaves

Directions:

1. Take a large glass bowl and your metal, electric mixer and set them in the refrigerator so they can chill.
2. In a separate bowl, add the yogurt and set that in the fridge.
3. Zest the lemon into a medium bowl that is microwavable.
4. Cut the lemon in half and then squeeze 1 tablespoon of lemon juice into the bowl.
5. Combine the cornstarch and water. Mix the ingredients thoroughly.
6. Pour in the honey and whisk the ingredients together.

7. Put the mixture into the microwave for 1 minute on high.
8. Once the microwave stops, remove the mixture and stir.
9. Set it back into the microwave for 15 to 30 seconds or until the mixture starts to bubble and thicken.
10. Take the bowl of yogurt from the fridge and pour in the warm mixture while whisking.
11. Put the yogurt mixture back into the fridge.
12. Take the large bowl and beaters out of the fridge.
13. Put your electronic mixer together and pour the whipped cream into the chilled bowl.
14. Beat the cream until soft peaks start to form. This can take up to 3 minutes, depending on how fresh your cream is.
15. Remove the yogurt from the fridge.
16. Fold the yogurt into the cream using a rubber spatula. Remember to lift and turn the mixture so it doesn't deflate.
17. Place back into the fridge until you are serving the dessert or for 15 minutes. The dessert should not be in the fridge for longer than 1 hour.
18. When you serve the lemony goodness, you will spoon it into four dessert dishes and drizzle with extra honey or even melt some chocolate to drizzle on top.
19. Add a little fresh mint and enjoy!

Nutritional facts: calories: 241, fats: 16 grams, carbohydrates: 21 grams, protein: 7 grams.

Cherry Brownies With Walnuts

Time: 25 to 30 minutes

Servings: 9

Ingredients:

- 9 fresh cherries that are stemmed and pitted or 9 frozen cherries
- ½ cup sugar or sweetener substitute
- ¼ cup extra virgin olive oil
- 1 teaspoon vanilla extract
- ¼ teaspoon sea salt
- ½ cup whole-wheat pastry flour
- ¼ teaspoon baking powder
- ⅓ cup walnuts, chopped
- 2 eggs
- ½ cup plain Greek yogurt
- ⅓ cup cocoa powder, unsweetened

Directions:

1. Make sure one of the metal racks in your oven is set in the middle.
2. Turn the temperature on your oven to 375 degrees Fahrenheit.
3. Using cooking spray, grease a 9-inch square pan.
4. Take a large bowl and add the oil and sugar or sweetener substitute. Whisk the ingredients well.
5. Add the eggs and use a mixer to beat the ingredients together.
6. Pour in the yogurt and continue to beat the mixture until it is smooth.

7. Take a medium bowl and combine the cocoa powder, flour, sea salt, and baking powder by whisking them together.
8. Combine the powdered ingredients into the wet ingredients and use your electronic mixer to incorporate the ingredients together thoroughly.
9. Add in the walnuts and stir.
10. Pour the mixture into the pan.
11. Sprinkle the cherries on top and push them into the batter. You can use any design, but it is best to make three rows and three columns with the cherries. This ensures that each piece of the brownie will have one cherry.
12. Put the batter into the oven and turn your timer to 20 minutes.
13. Check that the brownies are done using the toothpick test before removing them from the oven. Push the toothpick into the middle of the brownies and once it comes out clean, remove the brownies.
14. Let the brownies cool for 5 to 10 minutes before cutting and serving.

Nutritional facts: calories: 225, fats: 10 grams, carbohydrates: 30 grams, protein: 5 grams.

Stuffed Figs

Time: 20 minutes

Servings: 6

Ingredients:

- 10 halved fresh figs
- 20 chopped almonds
- 4 ounces goat cheese, divided
- 2 tablespoons of raw honey

Directions:

1. Turn your oven to broiler mode and set it to a high temperature.
2. Place your figs, cut side up, on a baking sheet. If you like to place a piece of parchment paper on top you can do this, but it is not necessary.
3. Sprinkle each fig with half of the goat cheese.
4. Add a tablespoon of chopped almonds to each fig.
5. Broil the figs for 3 to 4 minutes.
6. Take them out of the oven and let them cool for 5 to 7 minutes.
7. Sprinkle with the remaining goat cheese and honey.

Nutritional facts: calories: 209, fats: 9 grams, carbohydrates: 26 grams, protein: 8 grams.

Melon With Ginger

Time: 10 to 15 minutes

Servings: 4

Ingredients:

- ½ cantaloupe, cut into 1-inch chunks
- 2 cups of watermelon, cut into 1-inch chunks
- 2 cups honeydew melon, cut into 1-inch chunks
- 2 tablespoons of raw honey

- Ginger, 2 inches in size, peeled, grated, and preserve the juice

Directions:

1. In a large bowl, combine your cantaloupe, honeydew melon, and watermelon. Gently mix the ingredients.
2. Combine the ginger juice and stir.
3. Drizzle on the honey, serve, and enjoy! You can also chill the mixture for up to an hour before serving.

Nutritional facts: calories: 91, fats: 0 grams, carbohydrates: 23 grams, protein: 1 gram.

Chia Pudding With Strawberries

Time: 4 hours 5 minutes

Servings: 4

Ingredients:

- 2 cups unsweetened almond milk
- 1 tablespoon vanilla extract
- 2 tablespoons raw honey
- ¼ cup chia seeds
- 2 cups fresh and sliced strawberries

Directions:

1. In a medium bowl, combine the honey, chia seeds, vanilla, and unsweetened almond milk. Mix well.
2. Set the mixture in the refrigerator for at least 4

hours.

3. When you serve the pudding, top it with strawberries. You can even create a design in a glass serving bowl or dessert dish by adding a little pudding on the bottom, a few strawberries, top the strawberries with some more pudding, and then top the dish with a few strawberries.

Nutritional facts: calories: 108, fats: 4 grams, carbohydrates: 17 grams, protein: 3 grams.

Peaches With Blue Cheese Cream

Time: 20 hours 10 minutes

Servings: 4

Ingredients:

- 4 peaches
- 1 cinnamon stick
- 4 ounces sliced blue cheese
- ⅓ cup orange juice, freshly squeezed is best
- 3 whole cloves
- 1 teaspoon of orange zest, taken from the orange peel
- ¼ teaspoon cardamom pods
- ⅔ cup red wine
- 2 tablespoons honey, raw or your preferred variety
- 1 vanilla bean
- 1 teaspoon allspice berries
- 4 tablespoons dried cherries

Directions:

1. Set a saucepan on top of your stove range and add the cinnamon stick, cloves, orange juice, cardamom, vanilla, allspice, red wine, and orange zest. Whisk the ingredients well.
2. Add your peaches to the mixture and poach them for 2 hours or until they become soft.
3. Take a spoon to remove the peaches and boil the rest of the liquid to make the syrup. You want the liquid to reduce itself by at least half.
4. While the liquid is boiling, combine the dried cherries, blue cheese, and honey into a bowl.
5. Once your peaches are cooled, slice them into halves.
6. Top each peach with the blue cheese mixture and then drizzle the liquid onto the top.
7. Serve and enjoy!

Nutritional facts: calories: 211, fats: 24 grams, carbohydrates: 15 grams, protein: 6 grams.

Mediterranean Blackberry Ice Cream

Time: 15 minutes and time to chill

Servings: 6

Ingredients:

- 3 egg yolks
- 1 container of Greek yogurt
- 1 pound mashed blackberries
- ½ teaspoon vanilla essence
- 1 teaspoon arrowroot powder

- ¼ teaspoon ground cloves
- 5 ounces sugar or sweetener substitute
- 1 pound heavy cream

Directions:

1. In a small bowl, add the arrowroot powder and egg yolks. Whisk or beat them with an electronic mixture until they are well combined.
2. Set a saucepan on top of your stove and turn your heat to medium.
3. Add the heavy cream and bring it to a boil.
4. Turn off the heat and add the egg mixture into the cream through folding.
5. Turn the heat back on to medium and pour in the sugar. Cook the mixture for 10 minutes or until it starts to thicken.
6. Remove the mixture from heat and place it in the fridge so it can completely cool. This should take about one hour.
7. Once the mixture is cooled, add in the Greek yogurt, ground cloves, blackberries, and vanilla by folding in the ingredients.
8. Transfer the ice cream into a container and place it in the freezer for at least two hours.
9. Serve and enjoy!

Nutritional facts: calories: 402, fats: 20 grams, carbohydrates: 52 grams, protein: 8 grams.

Almond Shortbread Cookies

Time: 25 minutes and any time it takes to chill

Servings: 16 cookies

Ingredients:

- ½ cup coconut oil
- 1 teaspoon vanilla extract
- 2 egg yolks
- 1 tablespoon brandy
- 1 cup powdered sugar
- 1 cup finely ground almonds
- 3 ½ cups cake flour
- ½ cup almond butter
- 1 tablespoon water or rose flower water

Directions:

1. In a large bowl, combine the coconut oil, powdered sugar, and butter. If the butter is not soft, you want to wait until it softens up. Use an electric mixer to beat the ingredients together at high speed.
2. In a small bowl, add the egg yolks, brandy, water, and vanilla extract. Whisk well.
3. Fold the egg yolk mixture into the large bowl.
4. Add the flour and almonds. Fold and mix with a wooden spoon.
5. Place the mixture into the fridge for at least 1 hour and 30 minutes.
6. Preheat your oven to 325 degrees Fahrenheit.
7. Take the mixture, which now looks like dough, and divide it into 1-inch balls.
8. With a piece of parchment paper on a baking sheet,

arrange the cookies and flatten them with a fork or your fingers.
9. Place the cookies in the oven for 13 minutes, but watch them so they don't burn.
10. Transfer the cookies onto a rack to cool for a couple of minutes before enjoying!

Nutritional facts: calories: 250, fats: 14 grams, carbohydrates: 30 grams, protein: 3 grams.

Fruit Dip

Time: 10 to 15 minutes

Servings: 10

Ingredients:

- ¼ cup coconut milk, full-fat is best
- ¼ cup vanilla yogurt
- ⅓ cup marshmallow creme
- 1 cup cream cheese, set at room temperature
- 2 tablespoons maraschino cherry juice

Directions:

1. In a large bowl, add the coconut milk, vanilla yogurt, marshmallow creme, cream cheese, and cherry juice.
2. Using an electric mixer, set to low speed and blend the ingredients together until the fruit dip is smooth.
3. Serve the dip with some of your favorite fruits and enjoy!

Nutritional facts: calories: 110, fats: 11 grams, carbohydrates: 3 grams, protein: 3 grams.

Snacks

Baked Apples Mediterranean Style

Time: 25 minutes

Servings: 4

Ingredients:

- ½ lemon, squeezed for juice
- 1 ½ pounds of peeled and sliced apples
- ¼ teaspoon cinnamon

Directions:

1. Set the temperature of your oven to 350 degrees Fahrenheit so it can preheat.
2. Take a piece of parchment paper and lay on top of a baking pan.
3. Combine your lemon juice, cinnamon, and apples into a medium bowl and mix well.
4. Pour the apples onto the baking pan and arrange them so they are not doubled up.
5. Place the pan in the oven and set your timer to 25 minutes. The apples should be tender but not mushy.
6. Remove from the oven, plate and enjoy!

Nutritional facts: calories: 90, fats: 0.3 grams, carbohydrates: 24 grams, protein: 0.5 grams.

Fig-Pecan Energy Bites

Time: 20 minutes

Servings: 6

Ingredients:

- ½ cup chopped pecans
- 2 tablespoons honey
- ¾ cup dried figs, about 6 to 8, diced
- 2 tablespoons wheat flaxseed
- ¼ cup quick oats
- 2 tablespoons regular or powdered peanut butter

Directions:

1. Combine the figs, quick oats, pecans, peanut butter, and flaxseed into a bowl. Stir the ingredients well.
2. Drizzle honey onto the ingredients and mix everything with a wooden spoon. Do your best to press all the ingredients into the honey as you are stirring. If you start to struggle because the mixture is too sticky, set it in the freezer for 3 to 5 minutes.
3. Divide the mixture into four sections.
4. Take a wet rag and get your hands damp. You don't want them too wet or they won't work well with the mixture.
5. Divide each of the four sections into 3 separate sections.

6. Take one of the three sections and roll them up. Repeat with each section so you have a dozen energy bites once you are done.
7. If you want to firm them up, you can place them into the freezer for a few minutes. Otherwise, you can enjoy them as soon as they are little energy balls.
8. To store them, you'll want to keep them in a sealed container and set them in the fridge. They can be stored for about a week.

Nutritional facts: calories: 157, fats: 6 grams, carbohydrates: 26 grams, protein: 3 grams.

Frozen Blueberry Yogurt

Time: 30 minutes

Servings: 6

Ingredients:

- ⅔ cup honey
- 2 cups chilled yogurt
- 1 pint fresh blueberries
- 1 juiced and zested lime or lemon. You can even substitute an orange if your tastes prefer.

Directions:

1. With a saucepan on your burner set to medium heat, add the honey, juiced fruit, zest, and blueberries.

2. Stir the mixture continuously as it begins to simmer for 15 minutes.
3. When the liquid is nearly gone, pour the contents into a bowl and place in the fridge for several minutes. You will want to stir the ingredients and check to see if they are chilled.
4. Once the fruit is chilled, combine with the yogurt.
5. Mix until the ingredients are well incorporated and enjoy.

Nutritional facts: calories: 233, fats: 3 grams, carbohydrates: 52 grams, protein: 3.5 grams.

Strawberry Popsicle

Time: 10 minutes

Servings: 5

Ingredients:

- ½ cup almond milk
- 1 ½ cups fresh strawberries

Directions:

1. Using a blender or hand mixer, combine the almond milk and strawberries thoroughly in a bowl.
2. Using popsicle molds, pour the mixture into the molds and place the sticks into the mixture.
3. Set in the freezer for at least 4 hours.
4. Serve and enjoy—especially on a hot day!

Nutritional information: calories: 35, fats: 0.5 grams, carbohydrates: 7 grams, protein: 0.6 grams.

Chunky Monkey Trail Mix

Time: 1 hour 30 minutes

Servings: 6 cups

Ingredients:

- 1 cup cashews, halved
- 2 cups raw walnuts, chopped or halved
- ⅓ cup coconut sugar
- 1 cup coconut flakes, unsweetened and make sure you have big flakes and not shredded
- 6 ounces dried banana slices
- 1 ½ teaspoons coconut oil at room temperature
- 1 teaspoon vanilla extract
- ½ cup of chocolate chips

Directions:

1. Turn your crockpot to high and add the cashews, walnuts, vanilla, coconut oil, and sugar. Combine until the ingredients are well mixed and then cook for 45 minutes.
2. Reduce the temperature on your crockpot to low.
3. Continue to cook the mixture for another 20 minutes.
4. Place a piece of parchment paper on your counter.
5. Once the mix is done cooking, remove it from the crockpot and set on top of the parchment paper.
6. Let the mixture sit and cool for 20 minutes.
7. Pour the contents into a bowl and add the dried bananas and chocolate chips. Gently mix the

ingredients together. You can store the mixture in Ziplock bags for a quick and easy snack.

Nutritional facts: calories: 250, fats: 6 grams, carbohydrates: 18 grams, protein: 4 grams

Notes:

Chapter 10: Ten Tips for Success

Starting a diet is never easy. No matter how much you prepare and how dedicated you are when starting the diet, you will have moments when you struggle. These moments are harder when you feel that you don't have a support system or don't have the self-discipline to beat the cravings.

While this chapter is here to help you through your diet so you will be successful, it cannot stop you from having these moments. The truth is everyone has them from time to time, even people who have followed the diet for months. These tips are here to help you through these moments, give you advice, and make you realize that you are not alone. They're also here so you understand that these moments are okay. Even if you let yourself have a cheat day so you can let go of the intense cravings.

Tip 1: Be Proud of Yourself Everyday

It doesn't matter if this is your first day on the diet or your 100th, you need to be proud of yourself. Take a moment to smile and pat yourself on the back because you made it through the day. Look back on the day and think about the moments, if there were any, where you struggled. Even if you find yourself giving in to a craving, be proud of how long you tried to hold off on giving in to your craving.

One step to take to ensure you set aside time to be proud of yourself is to start a diet diary. Like a regular diary, you will write a passage every night, but you will focus on your diet. You will discuss anything you want to, such as what foods you ate, what you thought of them, any cravings you had, why you might have these cravings, and how they made you feel.

If you are having a particularly bad day, go back and read through some of your passages. Note other days where you felt the same way and read about your good days. Read your first passage and notice how far you've come since then.

Taking a moment to be proud of yourself, how far you've come, and why you want to continue following your goals will help you remain determined to continue the Mediterranean diet. Even if you're having a bad day, you will start to feel better. Furthermore, always remember that tomorrow is a new day.

Tip 2: Focus on Controlling Your Portions

One of the biggest tips that you can receive when starting a new diet, especially when you want to lose weight, is to look at your portions. In fact, watching your portions can help you lose weight without focusing heavily on a diet. The diet is an added benefit to your weight loss journey and health.

On the Mediterranean diet, your portions for common foods should look like this:

- ½ cup of pasta, rice, or other grains

- 1 cup of dry beans that are cooked
- 1 egg
- 2.1 ounces of meat, whether it is seafood or red meat
- 4.2 ounces of red or white wine
- 1 apple
- 1 orange
- 1 banana
- 7 ounces of melons, such as watermelon
- 1 ounce of grapes
- 1 ounce of nuts, whether it is included in a dish or as a snack
- 1 cup of milk
- 1 cup of yogurt
- 1 ounce of cheese
- 3.5 ounces of potatoes
- ½ cup of carrots
- ½ cup of cauliflower
- 1 cup of leafy greens

Tip 3: Make Time in Your Schedule to Focus on Your Meal Plan

Meal plans are an important part of your success, so you want to ensure you take time every week to create your meal plan, write up your grocery list, go grocery shopping, and even prepare any meals that you can. For example, you can start by baking any meat to place in the fridge for when you'll need it or by chopping your vegetables in advance.

Another way to help you make time is to plan and prepare your meals at the same time every week. You might play around with the days when you first start, but you'll find a time such as weekends or the middle of the week that is best for you. This can be a challenge for people who don't have a regular work schedule, so do your best. If you do need to change your days throughout the week, then make time to go through your upcoming week. Note when you have a few hours you can dedicate to meal planning, shopping, and meal preparations and write this down on your calendar.

Tip 4: Write Down Your Ideas

This might seem a little far-fetched to you as a beginner, but write down any ideas you have when it comes to meal planning, trying new recipes, or working on your meal prepping schedule. One way to do this is by keeping a journal so you can write down information as you're talking to other people about the topic or doing some research. You might also find yourself coming up with a new brilliant idea while you're driving to work. While you should pull over to write down the information, having a notebook next to you will keep you from forgetting your idea.

You can write down anything you want to. For instance, is there a certain ingredient that you really liked? Write it down and look for other recipes that include this specific ingredient. Keep your journal with you when you're cooking in the kitchen so you can write down information that will help you in the future, such as remembering to chop the vegetables the night before you make your casserole.

Tip 5: Always Keep Staple Foods in Your Kitchen

You already do this—you're running low on bread so you know you need to go to the store, or you know that your family goes through two loaves of bread in a week so you buy three. Keeping foods that are a staple for the Mediterranean diet in your kitchen will help you stay stocked up and give you enough food just in case you need to make a different meal one night. Some of the staple foods to keep while following the diet include whole wheat pasta, tofu, fish, whole grain rice, whole grain bread, oils, vegetables, eggs, fruit, nuts, and herbs.

Tip 6: Take Time to Eat

When you lead a busy life, it's easy to find yourself rushing through the meal. However, it's important to take time to eat. Stop rushing through your meal and enjoy the food that you made. Take a little longer to notice how the ingredients go together and what spices and herbs taste the best. If you have a family, this is the perfect opportunity to get some quality family time in before everyone goes their separate ways.

Another reason to eat slower is that you can lose weight by doing this. It takes your stomach several minutes to tell your brain that you are full. When you eat quickly, you'll become full minutes before your stomach tells your brain to stop eating, meaning you're eating so fast your brain doesn't have time to give you the feeling of fullness. Because it takes so long, you eat more than you should, and this causes your stomach to expand. But, when you eat slowly, you will know when you're full almost as soon as your stomach does.

Tip 7: You Don't Need to Prepare Every Meal

While you should write out every meal and all your snacks on your meal plan to help you stay on track, you don't need to prepare every meal in one or two days. Instead, look ahead to your week and notice when you are the busiest. For example, if you have a board meeting on Monday night and know that you won't be home until dinner time, this is a great night to prepare a meal in advance. This way, you can leave it in the fridge and warm it up once you get home. If you try to prepare every meal at the same time, you can start to feel overwhelmed and soon tell yourself that meal planning and preparation is more of a job than something fun to do. Feelings like these make it more likely that you'll give up on the task. Keep meal planning and preparing fun and you'll become more successful.

Tip 8: Let Your Food Cool Down All the Way Before Freezing

You know that food isn't supposed to sit on the counter for long or bacteria can start to grow in your meal. Because this is true, you'll want to place your food in the fridge to cool down. Once you make your soup or casserole, take it off the heat and let it cool down in an unsealed container in the fridge. If you put food in the freezer that isn't fully cool, you will change the texture and taste of the food.

Tip 9: Don't Skip Breakfast

It happens from time to time, you wake up late and don't have time to make the breakfast meal on your list. Because you don't want to grab sugary cereal or eat something unhealthy, you decide it's okay to skip breakfast as long as you eat lunch a little earlier. Instead, you need to stock your fridge with fruit as this will give you a quick breakfast if you can't make your egg or toast. Skipping breakfast will put your metabolism behind schedule, which makes it harder to lose weight, get the nutrients you need, and stay healthy.

Tip 10: Forgive Yourself

It's easy to add the wrong ingredient in a recipe or realize that the meal you made doesn't follow the Mediterranean diet like you thought. This is a common mistake for people, especially during the first couple of weeks on the diet. If you find out that you ate a meal that wasn't as

Mediterranean friendly as you thought, make a note and forgive yourself. You don't need to be perfect when it comes to the diet, you need to do your best. You will learn more about eating the Mediterranean way once you start the diet, which is why it's important to keep notes or a daily diary.

Notes:

Conclusion

You now know everything you need to know about meal planning on the Mediterranean diet. You even have several tips that will help you succeed on the diet and with your meal preparations. The key now is to do your best to work toward your goals and the things you want to accomplish on this diet.

You know the basics of the Mediterranean diet and what you'll need to do in order to stay on the diet. You also have 10 tips that will help you eat the Mediterranean way successfully.

Through the 4-week meal plan, you have a clear idea of how you can create a successful meal plan that not only follows the Mediterranean diet but also your schedule. For instance, you can prepare your meals in advance, so you don't need to worry about cooking something during your busiest weekdays.

Because there is a lot of information it can make you feel a bit overwhelmed, don't worry if you do as many people feel the same way. To help alleviate these feelings, I want to take you through the main takeaways of this book.

First, always take a moment throughout your day to be proud of the progress you've made when it comes to eating the Mediterranean way. Even if you made a mistake that day with your meal plan, take a moment to congratulate yourself. You are doing a great job and are on your way to becoming a successful Mediterranean dieter.

Second, following the Mediterranean food pyramid is the

simplest way to make sure you are eating the right foods. Most of the foods you should eat during the day consist of vegetables, fruits, herbs, oils, nuts, and seafood. You need to remember to limit your red meat and sweets to a very low number of servings during the month. In fact, the most you should have in one week is one serving.

Third, always take time during your week to plan your meals, create your shopping list, go grocery shopping, and prepare what meals you need to. This will help you stay on track with your diet. You don't need to make all your meals during the weekend, but looking ahead to see what days you are busy and preparing those meals will help you stay on your diet and give you an easier week.

Fourth, always remember to keep planning and prepping your Mediterranean meals fun. Try new meals at least once a week and make notes on what you liked and what you didn't.

Finally, think of following the Mediterranean diet as a lifestyle and not just a diet. When you start to incorporate the diet into your lifestyle, you will focus on becoming healthier throughout your day and not just when you are eating. Remember, one of the most important pieces of the Mediterranean food pyramid is that you need to exercise every day and save time for your family. These are two extremely important ingredients that will give you the best chance of success.

www.ingramcontent.com/pod-product-compliance
Lightning Source LLC
Chambersburg PA
CBHW071408210526
45465CB00001B/298